THE AMERICAN CATTLE DOCTOR

THE AMERICAN CATTLE DOCTOR

G. H. DADD, M.D.

VETERINARY PRACTITIONER

THE NECESSARY INFORMATION FOR PRESERVING THE HEALTH AND CURING DISEASES OF OXEN, COWS, SHEEP, AND SWINE

APPLEWOOD BOOKS
Bedford, Massachusetts

The American Cattle Doctor
was originally published in 1851.

Thank you for purchasing an Applewood Book.
Applewood reprints America's lively classics—books from the past that are still of interest to modern readers.
For a free copy of our current catalog, write to:

Applewood Books
P.O. Box 365
Bedford, MA 01730
www.awb.com

ISBN 978-1-55709-183-3

MANUFACTURED IN THE U.S.A.

Prepared for publishing by HP

THE AMERICAN CATTLE DOCTOR;

CONTAINING

THE NECESSARY INFORMATION

FOR

PRESERVING THE HEALTH AND CURING THE DISEASES

OF

OXEN, COWS, SHEEP, AND SWINE.

WITH

A GREAT VARIETY OF ORIGINAL RECIPES,

AND

VALUABLE INFORMATION IN REFERENCE TO

FARM AND DAIRY MANAGEMENT;

WHEREBY

EVERY MAN CAN BE HIS OWN CATTLE DOCTOR.

THE PRINCIPLES TAUGHT IN THIS WORK ARE, THAT ALL MEDICATION SHALL BE SUBSERVIENT TO NATURE; THAT ALL MEDICINAL AGENTS MUST BE SANATIVE IN THEIR OPERATION, AND ADMINISTERED WITH A VIEW OF AIDING THE VITAL POWERS, INSTEAD OF DEPRESSING, AS HERETOFORE, WITH THE LANCET AND POISON.

BY

G. H. DADD, M. D., VETERINARY PRACTITIONER,

AUTHOR OF "ANATOMY AND PHYSIOLOGY OF THE HORSE."

NEW-YORK:

ORANGE JUDD & COMPANY.

245 BROADWAY.

CONTENTS.

SHEEP.

SWINE.

APPENDIX.

INTRODUCTION.

THERE is no period in the history of the United States when our domestic animals have ranked so high as at the present time; yet there is no subject on which there is such a lamentable want of knowledge as the proper treatment of their diseases.

Governor Briggs, in a recent letter to the author, says, "You have my thanks, and, in my opinion, are entitled to the thanks of the community, for entering upon this important work. While the subject has engaged the attention of scientific men in other countries, it has been too long neglected in our own. Cruelty and ignorance have marked our treatment to diseased animals. Ignorant himself both of the disease and the remedy, the owner has been in the habit of administering the popular remedy of every neighbor who had no better powers of knowing what should be done than himself, until the poor animal, if the disease would not have proved fatal, is left alone, until death, with a friendly hand, puts a period to his sufferings: he is, however, often destroyed by the amount or destructive character of the remedies, or else by the cruel mode of administering them. I am persuaded that the community will approve of your exertions, and find it to their interest to support and sustain your system."

The author has labored for several years to substitute a safer and a more efficient system of medication in the treatment of diseased animals, and at the same time to point out to the American people the great benefits they will derive from the diffusion of veterinary education.

That many thousands of our most valuable cattle die under the treatment, which consists of little else than blood-letting, purging, and blistering, no one will deny; and these dangerous and destructive agents are frequently administered by men who are totally unacquainted with the nature of the agents they prescribe. But a better day is dawning; veterinary information is loudly called for — demanded; and the farmers will have it; *but it must be a safer and a more efficient system than that heretofore practised.*

The object of the veterinary art is not only congenial with human medicine, but the very same paths that lead to a knowledge of the diseases of man lead also to a knowledge of those of brutes.

Our domestic animals deserve consideration at our hands. We have tried all manner of experiments on them for the benefit of science; and science and scientific men should do something to repay the debt, by alleviating their sufferings and improving their condition. We are told that physicians of all ages have applied themselves to the dissection of animals, and that it was by analogy that those of Greece and Rome judged of the structure of the human body. For example, the Greeks and Arabians confined themselves to the dissection of apes and other quadrupeds. Galen has given us the anatomy of the ape for that of man; and it is clear that his dissections were restricted to brutes, when he says, that "if learned physicians have been guilty of gross errors, it is because they neglected to dissect animals." We advocate the establishment of veterinary schools, and the cultivation of our reformed system of veterinary medicine, on the broad principles of humanity. These poor animals are as susceptible to pain and suffering as we are. Has not the Almighty given us dominion over them, and placed them under our protection? Have we done our duty by them? Can we render a good account of our stewardship?

In almost every department of science the spirit of inquiry is abroad, investigation is active; yet, in this department, every thing is left to chance and ignorance. Men of all professions find it for their interest to protect property. The merchant, previous to sending his vessel on a voyage to a distant port, seeks out a skilful navigator to pilot that vessel into her desired haven with safety. He protects his property. We protect our property against the ravages of fire by insurance — we defend our houses from the lightning by conducting that fluid down the sides of the building into the earth. And shall we not protect our animals? Is not property invested in live stock as valuable, in proportion, as that invested in real estate? Can we permit live stock to degenerate and die prematurely from a want of knowledge of the fundamental laws of their being? Can we look on and see their heart's blood drawn from them — their flesh setoned, burned, and blistered — simply because it was the misguided custom of our ancestors?

We appeal to the American people at large. They have great encouragement to educate young men in this important branch of study; for the beneficial results will be, that the diseases of all classes of domestic animals will be better understood, and the great losses which this country sustains will, in a few years, be materially diminished. This is not all. The value of live stock will be increased at least twenty-five per cent!

Look for a moment at the amount of capital invested in live stock; and from these statistics the reader will perceive that not only the farmers, but the whole nation, will be enriched. There are in the United States at least 6,000,000 horses and mules; these, at the rate of $50 per head, amount to $300,000,000. It is also estimated that there are 20,000,000 of neat cattle; reckon these at $25 per head, and we get the snug little sum of $500,000,000. We have also 20,000,000 sheep. worth the same number of dollars. The number of swine have been computed at 24,000,000; and these, at $3 per head, give us $72,000,000. Hence the reader will see that the capital invested in this class of live stock reaches the enormous sum of $892,000,000. Add the 25 per cent. just alluded to, and we get a clear gain of $223,000,000. This sum would be sufficient to build veterinary schools and colleges capable of affording ample accommodations to every farmer's son in the Union. Hence we entreat the farming community to ponder on these subjects. They have only to say the word, and schools for the dissemination of veterinary information shall spring up in every section of the Union.

Does the reader wish to know how the *farmers* can accomplish this important object? We answer, there are four millions of men engaged in agricultural pursuits. Their number is three times greater than that of those engaged in navigation, the learned professions, commerce, and manufactures. Hence they have the numerical power to control the government of these United States, and of course can plead their own cause in the halls of congress, and vote their own supplies for educational purposes.

When the author first commenced a warfare against the lancet and other destructive agents, his only hopes of success were based on the coöperation of this mighty host of husbandmen; he well knew that there were many prejudices to be overcome, and none greater than those existing among his brethren of the same profession. The farmers have just begun to see the absurdity of bleeding an animal to death, with a view of saving life; or pouring down their throats powerful and destructive agents, with a view of making one disease to cure another! If the cattle doctors, then, will not reform, they must be reformed through the giant influence of popular opinion. Already the cry is, and it emanates from some of the most influential agriculturists in the country, — "*No more blood-letting!*" "*Use your poisons on yourselves.*"

To the cattle-rearing interest, at the hands of many of whom the author has received aid and encouragement, the following pages are dedicated; they are intended to furnish them with practical information, with a view of preventing disease, increasing the value of their stock, and restoring them to health when sick.

In reference to our reformed system of veterinary medication, it will be sufficient, in the present place, just to glance at the fundamental principles. In the succeeding pages these principles will be more fully explained. We contemplate the animal system as a complicated piece of mechanism, subject to the uncompromising and immutable laws of nature, as they are written upon the face of animate nature by the finger of Omnipotence.

All our intentions of cure being in accordance with nature's laws, (viz., promoting the integrity of the living powers,) we have termed our system a *physiological* one, though it is sometimes termed *botanic*, in allusion to the fact that most of our remedial agents are derived from the vegetable kingdom. We recognize a conservative or healing power in the animal economy, whose unerring indications we endeavor to follow; considering nature the physician, and the doctor her servant.

Our system proposes, under all circumstances, to restore the diseased organs to a healthy state, by coöperating with the vitality remaining in those organs, by the exhibition of sanative means, and, under all circumstances, to assist, and not oppose, nature in her curative processes. Poisonous substances, blood-letting, or processes of cure that act pathologically, cannot be used by us. The laws of animal life are physiological: they never were, nor ever will be, pathological.

The agents we use are just as we find them in the forest and the field, compounded by the Great Physician. Hence the reader will perceive that our aim is to depart from the popular debilitating and life-destroying practice, and approach as near as possible to the sanative.

G. H. D.

THE

AMERICAN CATTLE DOCTOR.

IMPORTANCE OF SUPPLYING CATTLE WITH PURE WATER.

In order to prevent many of the diseases to which cattle are liable, it is important that they be supplied with pure water. Cattle have often been known to turn away from the filthy fluid found in some troughs, which abound in slime and decayed vegetable matter; and, indeed, the common stagnated pond water is no better than the former. Such water has, in former years, proved itself to be a serious cause of disease; and, at the present day, death is running riot among the stock of our western, and also our northern farmers, when, to our certain knowledge, the cause exists, in some cases, under their very noses. The farmers ofttimes see their best stock sicken and die without any apparent cause; and the cattle doctors are running rough-shod through the *materia medica*, pouring down the throats of the poor brutes salts by the pound, castor oil by the quart; aloes, lard, and a host of kindred trash, follow in rapid succession, converting the stomach into a sort of apothecary's shop; setons are inserted in the "dewlap;" the horns are bored, and sometimes sawed off; and, as a last resort, the animals are blistered and bled. They sometimes recover, in spite of the violence done to the constitution; yet they drag out a low form of vitality, living it may be said, yet half dead, until some friendly epidemic puts a period to their sufferings.

The author's attention was first called to this subject on reading an article in an English work, the substance of which is as follows: A number of working oxen were put into a pasture, in which was a pond, considered to abound in good water. Soon after putting them there, they were attacked with scouring, upon which they were immediately removed to another field. The scouring continued. They still, however, drank at the same pond. They were shifted to another piece of very sweet pasture without arresting the disease. The farmer thought it evident that the pastures were not the cause of the disease; and, contrary to the advice of his friends, who affirmed that the spring was always noticed for the excellence of its water, fenced his pond round, so that the cattle could not drink; they were then driven to a distance and watered. The scouring gradually disappeared. The farmer now proceeded to examine the suspected pond; and, on stirring the water, he found it all alive with small creatures. He now stirred into the water a quantity of lime, and soon after an immense number of animalculæ were seen dead on the surface. In a short time, the cattle drank of this water without any injurious results.

There is no doubt but that inferior kinds of water produce derangement of the digestive organs, and subsequently loss of flesh, debility, &c. We have frequently made *post mortem* examinations of animals that have died from disease induced by debility, and have often found a large number of worms in the stomach and intestines, which, we firmly believe, had their origin either primarily from the water itself, or subsequently from its effects on the digestive function.

All decayed animal and vegetable matter tends to corrupt water, and render it unfit for the purposes of life. Now, if the farmer has the best spring in the world, and the water shall flow from it, as it sometimes does, through whole fields of gutter or dike, abounding in decayed filth, such water will be impregnated with agents that will more or less affect its purity.

REMARKS ON FEEDING CATTLE.

MANY of the most complicated diseases of cattle originate from the food: for example, it may be given in too large quantities — more than is needed to build up and repair the waste that is constantly going on. The consequence is, the animals get into a state of plethora, which is known by heaviness, dulness, unwillingness to move; there is a disposition to sleep, and they will lie down and often go to sleep in damp places. A chill of the extremities, or collapse of the capillaries, takes place, resulting in diseases of the lungs and pleura. At other times, if driven a short distance, and made to walk fast, they are liable to disease of the brain and other organs, which frequently terminates fatally.

The food may be of such a nature as shall be very difficult of digestion, such as cornstalks, foxgrass, frosted turnips, &c. The clover and grasses may abound in woody fibre, in consequence of being cut too late; they will then require more than the usual amount of gastric fluids to insalivate them, and more time to masticate, and, finally, extract their nutrimental properties. The stomach becomes overworked, producing sympathetic diseases of the brain and nervous structures. The stomach not being able to act on fibrous matter with the same despatch as on softer materials, the former accumulates in its different compartments, distends the viscera, interferes with the motion of the diaphragm, presses on the liver, seriously interfering with the bile-secreting process. In order to prevent the grass and clover from becoming tough and fibrous, it should be mowed early, and while in flower, and should be afterwards almost constantly attended to, if the weather is favorable; the more it is scattered about, the better will it be made, and the more effectually will its fragrance and other good qualities be preserved.

The food may also be deficient in nutriment. The effects of insufficient food are too well known to need much description: debility includes them all; it invades every function of the animal economy. And as life is the sum of the powers that resist disease, if disease is only the instrument of death it follows, of course, that whatever enfeebles life, or, in other words, produces debility, must predispose to disease.

Many cattle, during the winter, live on bad hay, which does not appear to contain any of that saccharine and mucilaginous matter which is found in good hay. When the spring comes, they are turned out to grass, and thus regain their flesh. Many, however, die in consequence of the sudden change.

It has been satisfactorily proved that fat cattle, of the best quality, may be produced by feeding them on boiled food.

Dr. Whitlaw says, "On one occasion, a number of cows were selected from a large stock, for the express purpose of making the trial: they were such as appeared to be of the best kind, and those that gave the richest milk. In order to ascertain what particular food would produce the best milk, different species of grass and clover were tried separately, and the quality and flavor of the butter were found to vary very much. But what was of the most importance, many of the grasses were found to be coated with silecia, or decomposed sand, too hard and insoluble for the stomachs of cattle. In consequence of this, the grass was cut and well steamed, and it was found to be readily digested; and the butter, that was made from the milk, much firmer, better flavored, and would keep longer without salt than any other kind. Another circumstance that attended the experiment was that, in all the various grasses and grain that were intended by our Creator as food for man or beast, the various oils that enter into their composition were so powerfully assimilated or combined with the other properties of the farinaceous plants, that the oil partook of the character of essential oil, and was not so easily evaporated as that of poisonous vegetables; and experience has proved that the same quantity of grass, steamed and given to the cattle, will produce more butter than when given in its dry state. This fact being established from numerous experiments, then there must be a great saving and superiority in this mode of feeding. The meat of such cattle is more wholesome, tender, and better flavored than when fed in the ordinary way." (For process of steaming, see Dadd's work on the Horse, p. 67.)

A mixed diet (boiled) is supposed to be the most economical for fattening cattle. "A Scotchman, who fattens 150 head of Galloway cattle, annually, finds it most profitable to feed with bruised flaxseed, boiled with meal or barley, oats or Indian corn, at the rate of one part flaxseed to three parts meal, by weight, — the cooked compound to be afterwards mixed with cut straw or hay. From four to twelve pounds of the compound are given to each beast per day." The editor of the Albany Cultivator adds, "Would it not be well for some of our farmers, who stall-feed cattle, to try this or a similar mode? We are by no means certain that the ordinary food (meaning, probably, bad hay and cornstalks) would pay the expense of cooking; but flaxseed is known to be highly nutritious, and the cooking would not only facilitate its digestion, but it would serve, by mixing, to render the other food palatable, and, by promoting the appetite and health of the animal, would be likely to hasten its thrift."

Mr. Hutton, who has long been celebrated for producing exceedingly fat cattle at a small cost, estimates that cost as follows: —

	s.	*d.*
"13 lbs. of linseed, bruised, or 2 lbs. per day for six days, and 1 lb. for Sunday, ...	1	9
32 lbs. of ground corn, or 5 lbs. per day for six days, and $2\frac{1}{2}$ lbs. for Sunday, at 1 d. per lb., ...	2	8
35 lbs. of turnips, given twice a day for six days, and thrice on Sunday, ...	1	6
Oats, $1\frac{1}{2}$ d.: labor on each beast, 6 d., ...		$7\frac{1}{2}$
Total cost of each beast per week, ...	6	$6\frac{1}{2}$

"The horses, cows, and young stock are also fed on this food, evidently with great advantage."

Mr. Workington, a successful dairyman, combining cut feed

and oil-cake with different sorts of green food, found that, by giving a middle-sized cow sixteen pounds of green food and two of boiled hay, with two pounds of ground oil cake, (*linseed would be preferable,*) and eight pounds of cut straw, the daily expense of her keep was only $5\frac{1}{2}$d., (about ten cents.) The oil-cake he found to be much more productive of milk when given with steamed food, than when employed without it. Varying their food from time to time is found to be of much more advantage to the cow; and this may probably arise from the additional relish with which the animal eats, or from the superior excitement of a new stimulus on the different secretions.

The following table represents the nutritive properties in each article of food:—

	Water.	Husk, or woody fibre.	Starch, gum, and sugar.	Gluten, albumen, &c.	Fatty matter.	Saline matter.
Oats, . . .	16	20	45	11	6	2.5
Beans, . .	14	8 to 11	40	26	2.5	3
Pease, . .	14	9	50	24	2.1	3
Indian corn,	14	6	70	12	5 to 9	1.5
Barley, . .	15	14	52	13.5	2 to 3	3
Meadow hay,	14	30	40	7.1	2 to 5	5 to 10
Clover hay,	14	25	40	9.3	3 to 5	9
Pea straw, .	10 to 15	25	45	12.3	1.5	4 to 5
Oat straw, .	12	45	35	1.3	0.8	6
Carrots, . .	85	3	10	1.5	0.4	1 to 2
Linseed, . .	9.2	8 to 9	35.3	20.3	20.0	6.3
Bran, . . .	13.1	53. 6	2	19.3	4.7	7.3

The most nutritious grasses are those which abound in sugar, starch, and gluten. Sugar is an essential element in the formation of good milk; hence the sweet-scented grasses are the most profitable to cultivate and feed to milch cows. At the same time, the farmer, if he does not, ought to know that large quantities of saccharine matter are extracted from clover and sweet grasses by the bees. Mr. White tells us that, "on a farm situated a few miles from London, the eldest son of the occupier had the management and profit of the bees given him, which induced him to increase the number of stocks beyond what had ever been kept on the farm before. It so happened that the sheep did not thrive so well as in former years, and on the farmer complaining at the cause to his man, as they had plenty of keep, the man replied, '*You will never have fat sheep so long as you suffer my young master to keep so many stocks of bees; they suck all the honey from the flowers, so that the clover is not half so nourishing, and does not produce half such good milk.*'" Had this man been acquainted with agricultural and animal chemistry, he would have had a clear conception of the seeming absurdity. All our labor or efforts to improve stock or crops will be fruitless, unless guided by chemical science. We must have sugar, starch, gluten, and other materials, to perfect animal organization. The animal may be in good health, the different functions free and unobstructed, and possess the power of reproducing the species; yet, if fed on substances which lack the materials necessary to the composition of bones, blood-vessels, and nerves, sooner or later its health becomes impaired. Reader, if you own cattle, and wish to preserve their health, give them boiled food occasionally; let them have their meals at regular hours, in sufficient quantity, and no more, unless they are intended for the butcher; then, an extra allowance may be given, with a view of fattening. They should be well littered, and the barns well ventilated; finally, keep them clean, avoid undue exposure, and govern them in a spirit of kindness and mercy.

THE BARN AND FEEDING BYRE.

It is well known that the more cleanly and comfortable cattle are kept, and the better the order in which their food is presented to them, the better they will thrive, and the more profitable they will be to the owner. Dr. Gunthier remarks, that "constant confinement to the barn is opposed to the nature of oxen, and becomes the source of numberless diseases. Endeavors are made to promote the lacteal secretion in cows, and the fattening of oxen, by means of heat: for this purpose, stables [barns] are converted into real stoves, either by not making them sufficiently large, or by crowding them to excess, or by preventing the access of air from without; and all this without recollecting that the skin, thus over-excited, must necessarily fall into a state of atony in a short time. Besides, the moist heat and the emanations of the dung cannot fail to exercise a destructive influence on the lungs and entire system. To these causes if we add the absolute want of exercise and the excess of food, we shall not be surprised at the number of diseases resulting from these different practices, and at the extraordinary forms which they ofttimes assume.

"Persons propose to themselves, by feeding in the barn, to augment the mass of dung; and the beasts are left in their excrement, sometimes up to the very knees. Seldom is there any care taken to cleanse their skin, and still less attention is directed to the feet. What wonder, then, if they exhibit so many forms of disease?"

The byre recommended by Mr. Lawson consists of two apartments—an inner apartment, or byre for feeding the cattle, and an outer apartment, or barn for containing the fodder. The byre is constructed at right angles with the barn, as follows: "At the distance of about three feet and a half from the side of the building, within, there are constructed, on the ground, in a straight line, a trough, having ten partitions for feeding ten animals. The troughs are so constructed, that there is a small and gradual declivity from the first or innermost to the last or outermost one; and the partitions separating them being made with a small arch at the bottom, a bucket of water, poured in at the uppermost, runs out at the last one through a spout in the wall; and a sweep of the broom carries off the whole remains of the food, rendering all the troughs quite clean and sweet. The whole food of the cattle is thus kept perfectly clean at all times.

"In a line with the feeding troughs, and immediately over them, runs a strong beam of wood, from one end of the byre to the other; which is strengthened by two strong upright supporters to the roof, placed at equal distances from the ends of the byre; and the main beam is again subdivided by the cattle stakes and chains, so as to keep each of the ten oxen opposite to his own feeding trough and stall.

"The three and a half feet of space between the troughs and outer wall, lighted by a glazed window, is the cattle feeder's walk, who passes along it in front of the cattle, and, with a basket, deposits before each of the cattle the food into the feeding trough of each. To prevent any of the cattle from choking on small pieces of turnips, &c., as they are very apt to do, the chains at the stakes are contrived of such a length, that no ox can raise his head too high when eating; for in this way, it is observed, cattle are generally choked.

"At the distance of about six feet eight inches from the feeding troughs, and parallel to them, is a dung grove and urine gutter. Here too, like the trough, there is a gradual declivity; so that the moment the urine passes from the cattle, it runs to the lowest end of the gutter, whence it is conveyed through the outer wall, in a spout, and deposited in the urinarium outside of the building. At this place is a large enclosed space, occupied as a compost dung-court. Here all sorts of stuff are collected for increasing the manure, such as fat, earth, cleanings of roads, ditches, ponds, rotten vegetables, &c.; and the urine from the byre, being caused to run over all these collected together, which is done very easily by a couple of wooden spouts, moved backwards and forwards to the urinarium at pleasure, renders the whole mass, in a short time, a rich compost dunghill; and this is done by the urine alone, which, in general, is totally lost. The dung of the byre, again, is cleared several times each day, and deposited in the dung-court. Along the edge of the dung-court a few low sheds are constructed, in which swine are kept, and these consume the refuse of the food.

"In the side wall of the byre, and opposite to the heads of the cattle, are constructed three ventilators; these are placed at the distance of about two feet four inches from the ground, in the inside of the byre, and pass out just under the roof. The inside openings of these are about thirteen inches in length, seven in breadth, and nine in depth; and they serve two good purposes. The breath of cattle being superficially lighter than atmospheric air, the consequence is, that in some byres the cattle are kept in a constant heat and sweat, because their breath and heat have no way to escape; whereas, by means of the ventilators, the air of the barn is kept in proper circulation, which conduces as much to the health of the cattle as to the preservation of the walls and timber of the byre, by drying up the moisture produced from the breath and sweat of the cattle, which is found to injure those parts of the building."

MILKING

The operation of milking should, if possible, always be performed by the same person, and in the most gentle manner; the violent tugging at the teats by an inexperienced hand is apt to make the animal irritable and uneasy during the operation, and unwilling to be milked. Many of the diseases of the teats and udder can be traced to violence done to the parts under the operation of milking. Young animals are often unwilling to be milked: here a little patience and kindness will perform wonders.

It is not the quantity of milk that gives value to the dairy cow; for the milk of one good cow will make more butter than that of two poor ones, each giving the same quantity of milk. Its most abundant principles are cream, caseous matter or curd, and whey. In these are also contained a saccharine matter, (sugar of milk,) muriate and phosphate of potassa, phosphate of lime, acetic acid, acetate of potassa, and a trace of acetate of iron. The three principal constituents (cream, curd, and whey) can easily be separated: thus the cream rises to the surface, and the curd and whey will separate if the milk becomes sour, or a little rennet is poured into it. When milk is intended to be made into cheese, no part of the cream should be separated. Good cheese is, consequently, rarely produced in those dairies where much butter is made; the former being robbed for the sake of the latter.

Sir J. Sinclair says, "If a few spoonfuls of milk are left in the udder of the cow at milking; if any of the implements used in the dairy are allowed to be tainted by neglect; if the dairy-house be kept dirty, or out of order; if the milk is either too hot or too cold at coagulation; if too much or too little rennet is put into the milk; if the whey is not speedily taken off; if too much or too little salt is applied; if butter is too slowly or too hastily churned; or if other minute attentions are neglected, the milk will be in a great measure lost. If these nice operations occurred once a month, or once a week, they might be easily guarded against; but as they require to be observed during every stage of the process, and almost every hour of the day, the most vigilant attention must be kept up during the whole season."

A KNOWLEDGE OF AGRICULTURAL AND ANIMAL CHEMISTRY IMPORTANT TO FARMERS.

It is a well-known fact that plants require for their germination and growth different constituents of soil, and that animals require different forms of food to build up the waste, and promote the living integrity — the vital powers.

In order to supply the materials necessary for animal and vegetable nutrition, we require alternate changes — the former in the diet, and the latter in the soil. Experience has proved that the cultivation of a plant for several successive years on the same soil impoverishes it, or the plant degenerates. On the contrary, if a piece of land be suffered to lie uncultivated for a short time, it will yield, in spite of the loss of time, a greater quantity of grain; for, during the interval of rest, the soil regains its original equilibrium. It has been satisfactorily demonstrated that a fruit-tree cannot be made to grow and bring forth good fruit on the same spot where another of the same species has stood; at least not until a lapse of years. This is a fact worth knowing, for it applies more or less to all forms of vegetation. Another fact of experience is, that some plants thrive on the same soil only after a lapse of years, while others may be cultivated in close succession, *provided the soil is kept in equilibrium by artificial means;* these are subsoiling, &c. Some kinds of plants improve the soil, while others impoverish or exhaust it. Professor Liebig tells us, "turnips, cabbages, beets, oats, and rye are considered to belong to the class which impoverish the soil; while by wheat, hops, madder, hemp, and poppies, it is supposed to be entirely exhausted." Many of our farmers expend large sums of money in the purchase of manure, with a view of improving the soil; and they suppose that their crops will be abundant in proportion to the amount of manure; yet many have discovered that, in spite of the extra expense and labor, the produce of their farms decreased.

The alternation of crops seems destined to effect a great change in agriculture. A French chemist informs us that the roots of plants imbibe matter of every kind from the soil, and thus necessarily abstract a number of substances, which are not adapted to the purposes of nutrition, and that they are ultimately expelled by the excretory vessels, and return to the soil as excrement. The excrementitious portion of the food also returns to the soil. Now, as excrement cannot be assimilated by the same animal or plant that ejected it, without danger to the organs of digestion or elimination, it follows that the more vegetable excrement the soil contains, the more unfitted must it be for plants of the same species; yet these excrementitious matters may, however, still be capable of assimilation by another kind of plant, which would absorb them from the soil, and render it again fertile for the first. In connection with this, it has been observed that several plants will flourish when growing beside each other; but it is not good policy to sow two kinds of seed together: on the other hand, some plants mutually prevent each other's development. The same happens if young cattle are suffered to graze and sleep in the barn together; the one lives at the expense of the other, which soon shows evidences of disease. The injurious effects of permitting young children to sleep with aged relatives are known to many of our readers; yet some parents see their children sicken and die without knowing the why or wherefore. From such facts as these,—which we might multiply to an indefinite extent, were it necessary,—we learn that nature's laws are immutable and uncompromising; and woe be to the man that transgresses them: they are a part of the divine law, which cannot be set at nought with impunity.

Ignorance on these important subjects has existed too long: yet we perceive in the distant horizon a ray of intellectual light, streaming through our schools and agricultural societies. The result will be, that succeeding generations will be better acquainted with nature's laws, from which shall flow untold blessings. Chemistry teaches us that animals and vegetables are composed of a vast number of different compounds, which are nearly all produced by the same elementary principles. Vegetables consist of carbon, hydrogen, and oxygen; and the same substances, with the addition of nitrogen, are the principal constituents of the animal economy. In a word, all the constituents of animal creation have actually been discovered in vegetables: this has, we presume, led to the conclusion that "all flesh is grass."

Many horticulturists complain that certain fruits and seeds have "*run out*," or degenerated. Has the stately oak, the elm, or the cedar degenerated? No. Each has preserved its identity, and will continue so to do, at least just as the Divine Artist intended they should, unless man, by his fancied improvements, interferes; and here, reader, permit us to ask if you ever knew a piece of nature's mechanism improved by human agency. Can we make a light better adapted to the wants of animate and inanimate creation than that which the sun, moon, and stars afford? Whenever we attempt to improve on immutable laws, as they are written on the face of creation, that moment we prevent the full and free play of these laws. Hence the practice of grafting scions of delicious fruit-trees on stock of an inferior order compromises its identity; and successive crops will show unmistakable evidences of encroachment. A son of the lamented Mr. Phinney tells us that he had some very fine sows, that he was desirous of breeding from, with a view of making "improvements." He bred in a close degree of relationship: in a short time, to use his own expression, "their sides appeared like two boards nailed together." Does the farmer wish to know how to prevent seeds and fruit "running out"? Let him study chemistry. Chemistry furnishes the information; it also teaches the husbandman the fact, that to put a plant, composed of certain essential elements, on a soil destitute of those elements, — or to graft a scion, requiring a certain amount of sap or juice, on a stock destitute of such sap or juice, expecting that they will germinate, grow to perfection, and preserve their identity, — would be just as absurd as to expect that a dry sow would nourish a sucking pig.

Agriculture being based on the equilibrium of the soils, a knowledge of chemistry is indispensable to every one who is desirous of keeping pace with the reforms of the age; for it is through the medium of that science alone that we are enabled to ascertain with certainty how this equilibrium is disturbed by the growth of vegetation. Then is it not a matter of deep interest to the farmer to know how this equilibrium is restored?

Does the farmer wish to know what kind of soil is necessary to nourish and mature a plant? Chemistry solves the problem. Does the farmer wish to know how to improve the soil? Let him refer to chemistry. Chemistry will teach the farmer how to analyze the soil; by that means he will learn which of the constituent elements of the plants and soil are constant, and which are changeable. By making an analysis of the soil at different periods, through the process of germination, growth, and maturity, we are enabled to ascertain the amount of excretory elements given out. Bergman tells us that he found, by analysis, in "100 parts of fertile soil, coarse silex 30 parts, silecia 30 parts, carbonate of lime 30 parts:" hence the fertility of the soil diminishes in proportion as one or the other of these elements predominates.

Ashes of wheat contain, among other elementary substances, 48 parts of silecia. Now, what farmer could expect to raise a good crop of wheat from a soil destitute of silecious earth, since this earth constitutes a large amount of the earthy part of wheat? There is no barrier to agricultural improvement so effectual as for farmers to continue their old customs purely because their forefathers did so. But prejudices are fast dying away before the rays of intellectual illumination; the farmers are fast seceding from the supposed infallibles of their forefathers, and will soon become "book" as well as practical husbandmen. "Book farming," assisted by practical knowledge, teaches that manures require admixture of milder materials to mitigate their force; for some of them communicate a disgusting or offensive quality to vegetables. They are charged with imparting a biting and acrimonious taste to radishes and turnips. Potatoes and grapes are known to borrow the foul taint of the ground. Millers observe a strong, disagreeable odor in the meal of wheat that grew upon land highly charged with the rotten recrements of cities. Stable dung is known to impart a disagreeable flavor to vegetables.

The same effects may be illustrated in the animal kingdom. Ducks are rendered so ill tasted from stuffing down garbage as sometimes to be offensive to the palate when cooked. The quality of pork is known by the food of the swine, and the peculiar flavor of water-fowl is rationally traced to the fish they devour. Thus a portion of the elements of manure and nutrimental matter passes into the living bodies without being entirely subdued. For example, we can alter the color of the cow's milk by mixing madder or saf fron in the food; the odor may be influenced by garlic; the flavor may be altered by pine and wormwood; and lastly, the medicinal effect may be influenced.

In the cultivation of grass the farmer will find it to his advantage to cultivate none but the best kinds; the whole pasture lands will then be filled with valuable grass seeds. The number of grass seeds worth cultivating is but few, and these should be sown separately. It is bad policy to sow different kinds of grass seed together—just as bad as to sow wheat, oats, turnips, and corn promiscuously.

The reason why the farmers, as a community, will be benefited by sowing none but the best seed is, because grass seeds are distributed through neighboring pastures by the winds, and there take root. Now, if the neighboring pastures abound in inferior grasses, the fields will soon be filled with useless plants, which are very difficult to be got rid of. We refer those of our readers who desire to make themselves acquainted with animal chemistry to Professor Liebig's work on that science.

ON BREEDING.

Large sums of money have, from time to time, been expended with a view of improving stock, and many superior cattle have been introduced into this country; yet, after a few generations, the beautiful form and superior qualities of the originals are nearly lost, and the importer finds to his cost that the produce is no better than that of his neighbors. What are the causes of this deterioration? We are told—and experience confirms the fact—that "like produces like." Good qualities and perfect organization are perpetuated by a union of animals possessing those properties: of course it follows, that malformation, hereditary taints, and vices are transmitted and aggravated.

The destructive practice of breeding "in and in," or, in

other words, selecting animals of the same family, is one of the first causes of degeneracy; and this destructive practice has proved equally unfortunate in the human family. Physical defects are the result of the intermarriage of near relatives. In Spain, the deformed and feeble state of the aristocracy arises from their alliances being confined to the same class of relatives through successive generations. But we need not go to Spain to verify such facts. Go into our churchyards and read on the tombstones the names of thousands of infants, — gems withered in the bud, — young men, and maidens, cut down and consigned to a premature grave; and then prove, if you can, that early marriages and near alliances are not the chief causes of this great mortality.

Mr. Colman, in an article on live stock, says, "There seems to be a limit beyond which no person can go. The particular breed may be altered and improved, but an entirely new breed cannot be produced; and in every departure from the original there is a constant tendency to revert back to it. The stock of the improved Durham cattle seems to establish this fact. If we have the true history of it, it is a cross of a Teeswater bull with a Galloway cow. The Teeswater or Yorkshire stock are a large, coarse-boned animal: the object of this cross was to get a smaller bone and greater compactness. By attempting to carry this improvement, if I may so call it, still further by breeding continually in and in, that is, with members of the same family, in a close degree of affinity, the power of continuing the species seems to become extinct; at least it approximates to such a result. On the other hand, by wholly neglecting all selection, and without an occasional good cross with an animal of some foreign blood, there appears a tendency to revert back to the large-boned, long-legged animal, from which the *improvement* began.

"There are, however, several instances of superior animals bred in the closest affinity; whilst, in a very great majority of cases, the failure has been excessive."

Overtaxing the generative powers of the male is another cause of deterioration. The reader is probably aware of the woful results attending too frequent sexual intercourse. If he has not given this subject the attention it demands, then let him read the records of our lunatic asylums: they tell a sad tale of woe, and prove to demonstration that, before the blast of this dire tornado, *sexual excess*, lofty minds, the suns and stars of our intellectual world, are suddenly blotted out. It spares neither age, sex, profession, nor kind. Dr. White relates a case which substantiates the truth of our position "The Prince of Wales, who afterwards became George the Fourth, had a stud horse of very superior qualities. His highness caused a few of his own mares to be bred to this stallion, and the produce proved every way worthy of the sire. This horse was kept at Windsor for public covering without charge, except the customary groom's fee of half a guinea. The groom, anxious to pocket as many half guineas as possible, persuaded all he could to avail themselves of the prince's liberality. The result was, that, being kept in a stable without sufficient exercise, and covering nearly one hundred mares yearly, the stock, although tolerably promising in their early age, shot up into lank, weakly, awkward, good-for-nothing creatures, to the entire ruin of the horse's character and sire. Some gentlemen, aware of the cause, took pains to explain it, proving the correctness of their statement by reference to the first of the horses got, which were among the best horses in England."

There is no doubt but that brutes are often endowed with extraordinary powers for sexual indulgence; yet, when kept for the purpose alluded to, without sufficient muscular exercise, — breathing impure air, and living on the fat of the farm, — his services in constant requisition, — then it is no wonder, that if, under these circumstances, the offspring are weak and inefficient.

Professor Youatt recommends that "valuable qualities once established, which it is desirable to keep up, should thereafter be preserved by occasional crosses with the best animals to be had of the same breed, but of a different family. This is the great secret which has maintained the blood horse in his great superiority."

The live stock of our farmers frequently degenerates in a very short space of time. The why and the wherefore is not generally understood; neither will it be, until animal physiology shall be better understood than it is at the present time. Men are daily violating the laws of animal organization in more ways than one, in the breeding, rearing, and general management of all kinds of domestic animals, — until the different breeds are so amalgamated, that, in many cases, it is a difficult task to ascertain, with any degree of certainty, their pedigree. If a farmer has in his possession a bull of a favorite breed, the neighboring stock-raisers avail themselves of his bullship's services by sending as many cows to him as possible: the consequence is, that the offspring got in the latter part of the season are good for nothing. The cow also, at the time of impregnation, may be in a state of debility, owing to some derangement in the organs of digestion; if so, impregnation is very likely to make the matter worse; for great sympathy exists between the organs of generation and those of digestion, and females of every order suffer more or less from a disturbed state of the stomach during the early months of pregnancy. In fact, during the whole stage they should be considered far from a state of health. Add to this the fact that impregnated cows are milked, (not generally, yet we know of such cases:) the fœtus is thus deprived of its due share of nourishment, and the extra nutrimental agents, necessary for its growth and development, must be furnished at the expense of the mother. She, in her turn, soon shows unmistakable evidences of this "robbing Peter to pay Paul" system, by her sunken eye, loss of flesh, &c., and often, before she has seen her sixth month of pregnancy, liberates the fœtus by a premature birth — in short, pays the penalty of disobedience to the immutable law of nature. On the other hand, should such a cow go safely through the whole period of gestation and parturition, the offspring will not be worth keeping, and the milk of the former will lack, in some measure, those constituents which go to make good milk, and without which it is almost worthless for making butter or cheese. A cow should never be bred from unless she shall be in good health and flesh. If she cannot be fatted, then she may be spayed. (See article *Spaying Cows.*) By that means, her health will improve, and she will be made a permanent milker. Degeneracy may arise from physical defects on the part of the bull. It is well known that infirmities, faults, and defects are communicated by the sexual congress to the parties as well as their offspring. Hence a bull should never be bred to unless he possesses the requisite qualifications of soundness, form, size, and color. There are a great number of good-for-nothing bulls about the country, whose services can be had for a trifle; under these circumstances, and when they can be procured without the trouble of sending the cow even a short distance, it will be difficult to effect a change.

If the farming community desire to put a stop to this growing evil, let them instruct their representatives to advocate the enactment of a law prohibiting the breeding to bulls or stallions unless they shall possess the necessary qualifications.

THE BULL.

Mr. Lawson gives us the following description of a good bull. It would be difficult to find one corresponding in all its details to this description; yet it will give the reader an idea of what a good bull ought to be. "The head of the bull should be rather long, and muzzle fine; his eyes lively and prominent; his ears long and thin; his horns white; his neck rising with a gentle curve from the shoulders, and small and fine where it joins the head; his shoulders moderately broad at the top, joining full to his chine and chest backwards, and to the neck-vein forwards; his bosom open; breast broad, and projecting well before his legs; his arms or fore thighs muscular, and tapering to his knees; his legs straight, clean, and very fine boned; his chine and chest so full as to leave no hollows behind the shoulders; the plates strong, to keep his belly from sinking below the level of his breast; his back or loin broad, straight, and flat; his ribs rising one above another, in such a manner that the last rib shall be rather the highest, leaving only a small space to the hips, the whole forming a round or barrel-like carcass; his hips should be wide placed, round or globular, and a little higher than the back; the quarters (from the hips to the rump) long, and, instead of being square, as recommended by some, they should taper gradually from the hips backwards; rump close to the tail; the tail broad, well haired, and set on so as to be in the same horizontal line with his back."

VALUE OF DIFFERENT BREEDS OF COWS.

Mr. Culley, in speaking of the relative value of long and short horns, says, "The long-horns excel in the thickness and firm texture of the hide, in the length and closeness of the hair, in their beef being finer grained and more mixed and marbled than that of the short-horns, in weighing more in proportion to their size, and in giving richer milk; but they are inferior to the short-horns in giving a less quantity of milk, in weighing less upon the whole, in affording less fat when killed, in being generally slower feeders, in being coarser made, and more leathery or bullish in the under side of the neck. In a few words, the long-horns excel in hide, hair, and quality of beef; the short-horns in the quantity of beef, fat, and milk. Each breed has long had, and probably may have, their particular advocates; but if I may hazard a conjecture, is it not probable that both kinds may have their particular advantages in different situations? Why not the thick, firm hides, and long, closer set hair, of the one kind be a protection and security against tempestuous winds and heavy fogs and rains, while a regular season and mild climate are more suitable to the constitutions of the short-horns? But it has hitherto been the misfortune of the short-horned breeders to seek the largest and biggest boned ones for the best, without considering that those are the best that bring the most money for a given quantity of food. However, the ideas of our short-horned breeders being now more enlarged, and their minds more open to conviction, we may hope in a few years to see great improvements made in that breed of cattle.

"I would recommend to breeders of cattle to find out which breed is the most profitable, and which are best adapted to the different situations, and endeavor to improve that breed to the utmost, rather than try to unite the particular qualities of two or more distinct breeds by crossing, which is a precarious practice, for we generally find the produce inherit the coarseness of both breeds, and rarely attain the good properties which the pure distinct breeds individually possess.

"Short-horned cows yield much milk; the long-horned give less, but the cream is more abundant and richer. The same quantity of milk also yields a greater proportion of cheese. The Polled or Galloway cows are excellent milkers and their milk is rich. The Suffolk duns are much esteemed for the abundance of their milk, and the excellence of the butter it produces. Ayrshire or Kyloe cows are much esteemed in Scotland; and in England the improved breed of the long-horned cattle is highly prized in many dairy districts. Every judicious selecter, however, will always, in making his choice, keep in view not only the different sorts and individuals of the animal, but also the nature of the farm on which the cows are to be put, and the sort of manufactured produce he is anxious to bring to market. The best age for a milch cow is betwixt four, or five, and ten. When old, she will give more milk; but it is of an inferior quality, and she is less easily supported."

METHOD OF PREPARING RENNET, AS PRACTISED IN ENGLAND.

Take the calf's maw, or stomach, and having taken out the curd contained therein, wash it clean, and salt it thoroughly, inside and out, leaving a white coat of salt over every part of it. Put it into an earthen jar, or other vessel, and let it stand three or four days; in which time it will have formed the salt and its own natural juice into a pickle. Take it out of the jar, and hang it up for two or three days, to let the pickle drain from it; resalt it; place it again in the jar; cover it tight down with a paper, pierced with a large pin; and let it remain thus till it is wanted for use. In this state it ought to be kept twelve months; it may, however, in case of necessity, be used a few days after it has received the second salting; but it will not be as strong as if kept a longer time. To prepare the rennet for use, take a handful of the leaves of the sweet-brier, the same quantity of rose and bramble leaves; boil them in a gallon of water, with three or four handfuls of salt, about a quarter of an hour; strain off the liquor, and, having let it stand until perfectly cool, put it into an earthen vessel, and add to it the maw prepared as above. To this add a sound, good lemon, stuck round with about a quarter of an ounce of cloves, which give the rennet an agreeable flavor. The longer the bag remains in the liquor, the stronger, of course, will be the rennet. The amount, therefore, requisite to turn a given quantity of milk, can only be ascertained by daily use and observation. A sort of average may be something less than a half pint of good rennet to fifty gallons of milk. In Gloucestershire, they employ one third of a pint to coagulate the above quantity.

MAKING CHEESE.

It is generally admitted that many dairy farmers pay more attention to the quantity than the quality of this article of food; now, as cheese is "a surly elf, digesting every thing but itself," (this of course applies to some of the white oak specimens, which, like the Jew's razors, were made to sell,) it is surely a matter of great importance that they should attend more to the quality, especially if it be intended for exportation. There is no doubt but the home consumption of good cheese would soon materially increase, for many thousands of our citizens refuse to eat of the miserable stuff "misnamed cheese."

The English have long been celebrated for the superior quality of their cheese; and we have thought that we cannot do a better service to our dairy farmers than to give, in as few words as possible, the various methods of making the different kinds of cheese, for which we are indebted to Mr. Lawson's work on cattle.

"It is to be observed, in general, that cheese varies in quality, according as it has been made of milk of one meal, or two meals, or of skimmed milk; and that the season of the year, the method of milking, the preparation of the rennet, the mode of coagulation, the breaking and gathering of the curd, the management of the cheese in the press, the method of salting, and the management of the cheese-room, are al objects of the highest importance to the cheese manufacturer and yet, notwithstanding this, the practice, in most of these respects, is still regulated by little else than mere chance or custom, without the direction of enlightened observation or the aid f well-conducted experiment.

GLOUCESTER CHEESE.

"In Gloucestershire, where the manufacture of cheese is perhaps as well understood as in any part of the world, they make the best cheeses of a single meal of milk; and, when this is done in the best manner, the entire meal of milk is used, without any addition from a former meal. But it not unfrequently happens that a portion of the milk is reserved and set by to be skimmed for butter; and at the next milking this proportion is added to the new milk, from which an equal quantity has been taken for a similar purpose. One meal cheeses are principally made here, and go by the name of *best making*, or simply *one meal cheeses*. The cheeses are distinguished into *thin* and *thick*, or *single* and *double*; the last having usually four to the hundred weight, (112 pounds,) the other about twice that number. The best double Gloucester is always made from new milk.

"The true single Gloucester cheese is thought by many to be the best, in point of flavor, of any we have. The season for making their thin or single cheese is mostly from April to November; but the principal season for the thick or double is confined to May, June, and the early part of July. This is a busy season in the dairy; for at an earlier period the milk is not rich enough, and if the cheese be made later in the summer, they do not acquire sufficient age to be marketable next spring. Very many cheeses, however, can be made even in winter from cows that are well fed. The cows are milked in summer at a very early hour; generally by four o'clock in the morning, before the day becomes hot, and the animals restless and unruly.

CHESTER CHEESE.

"After the milk has been strained, to free it from any impurities, it is conveyed into a cooler placed upon feet like a table, having a spigot at the bottom for drawing off the milk. This, when sufficiently cooled, is drawn off into pans, and the cooler again filled. In some cases, the cooler is large enough to hold a whole meal's milk at once. The rapid cooling thus produced (which, however, is necessary only in hot weather, and during the summer season) is found to be of essential utility in retarding the process of fermentation, and thereby preventing putridity from commencing in the milk before two meals of it can be put together. Some have thought that the cheese might be improved by cooling the evening's milk still more rapidly, and that this might be effected by repeatedly drawing it off from and returning it into the cistern. When the milk is too cold, a portion of it is warmed over the fire and mixed with the rest.

stand over night. The whole of this infusion is, in the morning, mixed with the milk in the cheese-tub, and the rag dipped in the milk and rubbed on the palm of the hand as long as any of the coloring matter can be made to come away.

"The next operation is salting; and this is done, either by laying the cheese, immediately after it comes out of the press, on a clean, fine cloth in the vat, immersed in brine, to remain for several days, turning it once every day at least; or by covering the upper surface of the cheese with salt every time it is turned, and repeating the application for three successive days, taking care to change the cloth twice during the time In each of these methods, the cheese, after being so treated, is taken out of the vat, placed upon the salting bench, and the whole surface of it carefully rubbed with salt daily for eight or ten days. If it be large, a wooden hoop or a fillet of cloth is employed to prevent renting. The cheese is then washed in warm water or whey, dried with a cloth, and laid on what is called the *drying bench*. It remains there for about a week, and is thence removed to the *keeping house*. In Cheshire, it is found that the greatest quantity of salt used for a cheese of sixty pounds is about three pounds; but the proportion of this retained in the cheese has not been determined.

"When, after salting and drying, the cheeses are deposited in the cheese-room or store-house, they are smeared all over with fresh butter, and placed on shelves fitted to the purpose, or on the floor. During the first ten or fifteen days, smart rubbing is daily employed, and the smearing with butter repeated. As long, however, as they are kept, they should be every day turned; and the usual practice is to rub them three times a week in summer and twice in winter.

STILTON CHEESE.

"Stilton cheese is made by putting the night's cream into the morning's new milk along with the rennet. When the curd has come, it is not broken, as in making other cheese, but taken out whole, and put into a sieve to drain gradually. While this is going on, it is gently pressed, and, having become firm and dry, is put into a vat, and kept on a dry board. These cheeses are exceedingly rich and valuable. They are called the Parmesan of England, and weigh from ten to twelve pounds. The manufacture of them is confined almost exclusively to Leicestershire, though not entirely so.

DUNLOP CHEESE.

"In Scotland, a species of cheese is produced, which has long been known and celebrated under the name of *Dunlop* cheese. The best cheese is made by such as have a dozen or more cows, and consequently can make a cheese every day; one half of the milk being immediately from the cow, and the other of twelve hours' standing. Their method of making it is simple. They endeavor to have the milk as near as may be to the heat of new milk, when they apply the rennet, and whenever coagulation has taken place, (which is generally in ten or twelve minutes,) they stir the curd gently, and the whey, beginning to separate, is taken off as it gathers, till the curd be pretty solid. When this happens, they put it into a drainer with holes, and apply a weight. As soon as this has had its proper effect, the curd is put back again into the cheese-tub, and, by means of a sort of knife with three or four blades, is cut into very small pieces, salted, and carefully mixed by the hand. It is now placed in the vat, and put under the press. This is commonly a large stone of a cubical shape, from half a ton to a ton in weight, fixed in a frame of wood, and raised and lowered by an iron screw. The cheese is frequently taken out, and the cloth changed; and as soon as it has been ascertained that no more whey remains, it is removed, and placed on a dry board or pine floor. It is turned and rubbed frequently with a hard, coarse cloth, to prevent moulding or breeding mites. No coloring matter is used in making Dunlop cheese, except by such as wish to imitate the English cheese

GREEN CHEESE.

"Green cheese is made by steeping over night, in a proper quantity of milk, two parts of sage with one of marigold leaves, and a little parsley, after being bruised, and then mixing the curd of the milk, thus *greened*, as it is called, with the curd of the white milk. These may be mixed irregularly or fancifully, according to the pleasure of the operator. The management in other respects is the same as for common cheese."

Mr. Colman says, "In conversation with one of the largest wholesale cheesemongers and provision-dealers in the country, he suggested that there were two great faults of the American cheese, which somewhat prejudiced its sale in the English market. He is a person in whose character and experience entire confidence may be placed.

"The first fault was the softness of the rind. It often cracked, and the cheese became spoiled from that circumstance.

"The second fault is the acridness, or peculiar, smart, bitter taste often found in American cheese. He thought this might be due, in part, to some improper preparation or use of the rennet, and, in part, to some kind of feed which the cows found in the pastures.

"The rind may be made of any desired hardness, if the cheese be taken from the press, and allowed to remain in brine, so strong that it will take up no more salt, for four or five hours. There must be great care, however, not to keep it too long in the brine.

"The calf from which the rennet is to be taken should not be allowed to suck on the day on which it is killed. The office of the rennet, or stomach of the calf, is, to supply the gastric juice by which the curdling of the milk is effected. If it has recently performed that office, it will have become, to a degree, exhausted of its strength. Too much rennet should not be applied. Dairymaids, in general, are anxious to have the curd 'come soon,' and so apply an excessive quantity, to which he thinks much of the acrid taste of the cheese is owing. Only so much should be used as will produce the effect in about fifty minutes. For the reason above given, the rennet should not, he says, be washed in water when taken from the calf, as it exhausts its strength, but be simply salted.

"When any cream is taken from the milk to be made into butter, the buttermilk should be returned to the milk of which the cheese is to be made. The greatest care should be taken in separating the whey from the cheese. When the pressing or handling is too severe, the whey that runs from the curd will appear of a white color. This is owing to its carrying off with it the small creamy particles of the cheese, which are, in fact, the richest part of it. After the curd is cut or broken, therefore, and not squeezed with the hand, and all the whey is allowed to separate from it that can be easily removed, the curd should be taken out of the tub with the greatest care, and laid upon a coarse cloth attached to a frame like a sieve, and there suffered to drain until it becomes quite dry and mealy, before being put into the press. The object of pressing should be, not to express the whey, but to consolidate the cheese. There should be no aim to make whey butter. All the butter extracted from the whey is so much of the proper richness taken from the cheese."

MAKING BUTTER.

It is a matter of impossibility to make a superior article of butter from the milk of a cow in a diseased state; for if either of the organs of secretion, absorption, digestion, or circulation, be deranged, we cannot expect good blood. The milk being a secretion from the blood, it follows that, in order to have good milk, we must have pure blood. A great deal depends also on the food; certain pastures are more favorable to the production of good milk than others. We know that many vegetables, such as turnips, garlic, dandelions, will impart a disagreeable flavor to the milk. On the other hand, sweet-scented grasses and boiled food improve the quality, and, generally, increase the quantity of the milk, provided, however, the digestive organs are in a physiological state.

The processes of making butter are various in different parts of the United States. We are not prepared, from experience, to discuss the relative merits of the different operations of churning: suffice it to say, that the important improvements that have recently been made in the construction of churns promise to be of great advantage to the dairyman.

The method of churning in England is considered to be favorable to the production of good butter. From twelve to twenty hours in summer, and about twice as long in winter, are permitted to elapse before the milk is skimmed, after it has been put into the milk-pans. If, on applying the tip of the finger to the surface, nothing adheres to it, the cream may be properly taken off; and during the hot summer months, this should always be done in the morning, before the dairy becomes warm. The cream should then be deposited in a deep pan, placed in the coolest part of the dairy, or in a cool cellar, where free air is admitted. In hot weather, churning should be performed, if possible, every other day; but if this is not convenient, the cream should be daily shifted into a clean pan, and the churning should never be less frequent than twice a week. This work should be performed in the coolest time of the day, and in the coolest part of the house. Cold water should be applied to the churn, first by filling it with this some time before the cream is poured in, or it may be kept cool by the application of a wet cloth. Such means are generally necessary, to prevent the too rapid acidification of the cream, and formation of the butter. We are indebted for much of the poor butter, (*cart-grease* would be a more suitable name,) in which our large cities abound, to want of due care in churning: it should never be done too hastily, but — like "Billy Gray's" drumming — well done. In winter the churn may be previously heated by first filling it with hot water, the operation to be performed in a moderately warm room.

In churning, a moderate and uninterrupted motion should be kept up during the whole process; for if the motion be too rapid, heat is generated, which will give the butter a rank flavor; and if the motion is relaxed, the butter will go back, as it is termed

WASHING BUTTER.

"When the operation is properly conducted, the butter, after some time, suddenly forms, and is to be carefully collected and separated from the buttermilk. But in doing this, it is not sufficient merely to pour off the milk, or withdraw the butter from it; because a certain portion of the caseous and serous parts of the milk still remains in the interstices of the butter, and must be detached from it by washing, if we would obtain it pure. In washing butter, some think it sufficient to press the mass gently between the hands; others press it strongly and frequently, repeating the washings till the water comes off quite clear. The first method is preferable when the butter is made daily, for immediate use, from new milk or cream; because the portions of such adhering to it, or mixed with it, contribute to produce the sweet agreeable flavor which distinguishes new cream. But when our object is to prepare butter for keeping, we cannot repeat the washings too often, since the presence of a small quantity of milk in it will, in less than twelve hours after churning, cause it sensibly to lose its good qualities.

"The process of washing butter is usually nothing more than throwing it into an earthen vessel of clear cool water, working it to and fro with the hands, and changing the water until it comes off clear. A much preferable method, however, and that which we believe is now always practised by those who best understand the business, is to use two broad pieces of wood, instead of the hands. This is to be preferred, not only on account of its apparently greater cleanliness, but also because it is of decided advantage to the quality of the butter. To this the warmth of the hand gives always, more or less, a greasy appearance. The influence of the heat of the hand is greater than might at first have been suspected. It has always been remarked, that a person who has naturally a warm hand never makes good butter."

COLORING BUTTER.

As butter made in winter is generally pale or white, and its richness, at the same time, inferior to that which is made during the summer months, the idea of excellence has been associated with the yellow color. Means are therefore employed, by those who prepare and sell butter, to impart to it the yellow color where that is naturally wanting. The substances mostly employed in England and Scotland are the root of the carrot and the flowers of the marigold. The juice of either of these is expressed and passed through a linen cloth. A small quantity of it (and the proportion of it necessary is soon learned by experience) is diluted with a little cream, and this mixture is added to the rest of the cream when it enters the churn. So little of this coloring matter unites with the butter, that it never communicates to it any peculiar taste.

DESCRIPTION OF THE ORGANS OF DIGESTION IN CATTLE.

Œsophagus, or *Gullet*. — This tube extends from the mouth to the stomach, and is the medium through which the food is conveyed to the latter organ. This tube is furnished with spiral muscles, which run in different directions. By this arrangement, the food ascends or descends at the will of the animal. The inner coat of the gullet is a continuation of the same membrane that lines the mouth, nostrils, &c. The gullet passes down the neck, inclining to the left side of the windpipe, until it reaches the diaphragm, through a perforation of which it passes, and finally terminates in the stomach. The food, having undergone a slight mastication by the action of the teeth, is formed into a pellet, and, being both moistened and lubricated with saliva, passes down the gullet, by the action of the muscles, and falls immediately into the paunch, or rumen ; here the food undergoes a process of maceration, or trituration. The food, after remaining in this portion of the stomach a short time, and being submitted to the united action of heat and moisture, passes into another division of the stomach, called *reticulum*, the inner surface of which abounds in cells : at the bottom, and indeed in all parts of them there are glands, which secrete from the blood the gastric fluids. This stomach possesses a property similar to that of the bladder, viz., that of contracting upon its contents. In the act of contracting, it squeezes out a portion of the partly masticated food and fluids ; the former comes within the spiral muscles, is embraced by them, and thus ascends the gullet, and passes into the mouth for remastication. The soft and fluid parts continue on to the manyplus and true digestive stomach. The second stomach again receives a portion from the paunch, and the process is continued.

Rumination and digestion, however, are mechanico-vital actions, and can only be properly performed when the animal is in a healthy state.

Now, a portion of the food, we just observed, had ascended

the gullet by the aid of spiral muscles, and entered the mouth; it is again submitted to the action of the grinders, and a fresh supply of saliva; it is at length swallowed a second time, and goes through the same routine as that just described, passing into the manyplus or manifolds, as it is termed.

The manyplus abounds internally in a number of leaves, called laminæ. Some of these are attached to the upper and lower portion of the division, and also float loose, and penetrate into the œsophagian canal. The laminæ have numerous projections on their surface, resembling the papillæ to be found on the tongue. The action of this stomach is one of alternate contraction and expansion: it secretes, however, like the other compartments of the stomach, its due share of gastric fluids, with a view not only of softening its contents, but for the purpose of defending its own surface against friction. The mechanical action of the stomach is communicated to it partly by the motion of the diaphragm, and its own muscular arrangement. It will readily be perceived, that by this joint action the food is submitted to a sort of grinding process. Hence any over-distention of the viscera, from either food or gas, will embarrass and prevent the free and full play of this organ. The papillæ, or prominences, present a rough and sufficiently hard exterior to grind down the food, unless it shall have escaped the reticulum in too fibrous a form: fox-grass, cornstalks, and frosted turnips are very apt to make sad havoc in this and other parts of the stomach, owing to their unyielding nature; for the stomach, like other parts of the organization, suffers from over-exertion, and a corresponding debility ensues.

The fourth division of the stomach of the ox is called *abomasum.* It somewhat resembles the duodenum of the horse in its function, it being the true digestive stomach. It is studded with numerous nerves, blood-vessels, and small glands. It is a laboratory admirably fitted up by the Divine Artist, and is capable of carrying on the chemico-vital process as long as the animal lives, provided its healthy functions are not impaired. The glands alluded to secrete from the blood a powerful solvent, called the *gastric juice,* which is the agent in reducing the food to chyme and chyle. This, however, is accomplished by the united agency of the bile and pancreatic juice. Both these fluids are conveyed into the abomasum by means of small tubes or canals. Secretions also take place from the inner membrane of the intestines, and, as the result of the united action of all these fluids, aided by the muscular motion just alluded to, which is also communicated to the intestines, a substance is formed called *chyle,* which is the most nutritious portion of the food, and has a milky appearance. The chyle is received into a set of very minute tubes, called *lacteals,* which are exceedingly numerous, and arise by open mouths from the inner surface of the abomasum and intestines. They receive the chyle; from thence it passes into a receptacle, and finally into the thoracic duct. The thoracic duct opens into a vein leading directly to the heart; so that whatever portion of the chyle is not actually needed by the organism is thoroughly mixed with the general mass of blood. That portion of chyme which is not needed, or cannot be converted into chyle, descends into the intestines, and is finally carried out of the body by the rectum.

The manner in which the gastric fluids act on alimentary matter, is by solution and chemical action; for cornstalks and fox-grass, that cannot be dissolved by ammonia or alcohol, yield readily to the solvent power of the gastric secretion. Bones and other hard substances are reduced to a pulpy mass in the stomach of a dog; while, at the same time, many bodies of delicate texture remain in the stomach, and ultimately are ejected, without being affected by the gastric fluids. This different action on different subjects is analogous to the operation of chemical affinity, and corroborates the theory that digestion is effected by solution and chemical action.

The Spleen, or *Milt,* is an oblong, dark-colored substance, having attachments to the paunch. It is composed of blood-vessels, nerves, and lymphatics, united by cellular structure. It appears to serve as a reservoir for the blood that may be designed for the secretion of bile in the liver. P. M. Rogesays, "Any theory that assigns a very important function to the spleen will be overturned by the fact, that in many animals the removal of this organ, far from being fatal, or interrupting, in any sensible manner, the continuance of the functions, seems to be borne with perfect impunity." Sir E. Home, Bichat, Leuret, Lassaigne, and others, suppose that "the spleen serves as a receptacle for the superfluous quantity of fluid taken into the stomach."

The Liver is a dense gland, of a lobulated structure, situated below the diaphragm, or "skirt." It is supplied, like other organs, with arterial blood, by vessels, called *hepatic* arteries, which are sent off from the great aorta. It receives also a large amount of venous blood, which is distributed through its substance by a separate set of vessels, derived from the venous system. The veins which receive the blood that has circulated in the usual manner unite together into a large trunk, called vena portæ, (gate vein,) and this vein, on entering the liver, ramifies like an artery, and ultimately terminates in the branches of the hepatic veins, which transmit the blood, in the ordinary course of circulation, to the vena cava, (hollow vein.) Mr. Kiernan says, "The hepatic veins, together with the lobules which surround them, resemble, in their arrangement, the branches and leaves of a tree, the substance of the lobules being disposed around the minute branches of the veins like the parenchyma of a leaf around its fibres. The hepatic veins may be divided into two classes, namely, those contained in lobules, and those contained in canals formed by lobules. The first class is composed of interlobular branches, one of which occupies the centre of each lobule, and receives the blood from a plexus formed in the lobule by the portal vein; and the second class of hepatic veins is composed of all those vessels contained in canals formed by the lobules, and including numerous small branches, as well as the large trunks terminating in the inferior cava. The external surface of every lobule is covered by an expansion of '*Glisson's capsule*,' by which it is connected to, as well as separated from, contiguous lobules, and in which branches of the hepatic duct, portal veins, and hepatic artery ramify. The ultimate branches of the hepatic artery terminate in the branches of the portal vein, where the blood they respectively contain is mixed together, and from which mixed blood the bile is secreted by the lobules, and conveyed away by the hepatic ducts. The remaining blood is returned to the heart by the hepatic veins, the beginnings of which occupy the centre of each lobule, and, when collected into trunks, pour their contents into the inferior cava. Hence the blood which has circulated through the liver, and has thereby lost its arterial character, is, in common with that which is returning from other parts, poured into the vena portæ, and contributes its share in furnishing materials for the biliary secretion. The hepatic artery furnishes nutrition to the liver itself."

The bile, having been secreted, accumulates in the gall-bladder, where it is kept for future use. When the healthy action of the fourth stomach is interrupted, the bile is supposed to be reabsorbed,—it enters into the different tissues, producing yellowness of the eyes; the malady is then termed *yellows*, *jaundice*, &c. Sometimes the passage of the bile is obstructed by calculi, or gall-stones; they have been found in great numbers in oxen.

The Pancreas is composed of a number of lobules or glands; a small duct proceeds from each; they unite and form a common canal, which proceeds towards, and terminates in, the fourth stomach. The pancreatic juice appears to be exceedingly analogous, both in its sensible properties and chemical composition, to the saliva.

"The recent researches of MM. Bouchardat, Sandras, Mialhe, Bareswil, and Bernard himself, have placed beyond a doubt the existence of a ferment, in some of the fluids which mix with the alimentary mass, destined to convert starchy matters into sugar. They have proved that the gastric juice has for its peculiar office the solution and digestion of azotized substances. There remained to be ascertained the real agent for the digestion of fatty matters; that is to say, the agent in the formation of chyle out of those substances.

"M. Bernard has proved that this remarkable office is performed by the pancreatic juice; he has demonstrated the fact by three conclusive proofs.

"1. The pancreatic juice, pure and recently formed, forms an emulsion with oils and fats with the greatest facility. This emulsion may be preserved for a long time, and the fatty substance soon undergoes a fermentation which separates its constituent acids.

"2. The chyle only begins to appear in the lacteals below that part of the intestinal tube where the pancreatic juice enters it to mix with the alimentary matters.

"3. In disorders of the pancreas, we find that the fatty matters, contained in the food, pass entire in the evacuations."

The above is an extract from the report of a body composed of several members of the French Academy of Sciences. "M. Bernard" (continues the report) "has exhibited to us the first of these experiments, and has furnished us with the means of repeating it with the several varieties of the gastric juice. We have not the slightest doubt on the subject. It is incontestable that fatty substances are converted into an emulsion by this juice, in a manner easy and persistent, and it is no less true that the saliva, the gastric juice, and the bile are destitute of this property.

"The second demonstration can be given in various modes; but the author has discovered, in the peculiar arrangement of the digestive apparatus of the rabbit, an unexceptional means of obtaining it with the greatest precision, and at will. The pancreatic juice enters the intestinal tube of this animal about fourteen inches below the point where the bile is poured in. Now, as long as the food is above the region where it mixes with the pancreatic juice, there appears to be no formation and separation of a milky chyle; nothing shows that the fatty matters are reduced to an emulsion. On the contrary, as soon as the pancreatic juice mixes with the alimentary matters, we observe the fat to be converted into an emulsion, and a milky chyle to fill the corresponding lacteals. Nothing can give an idea of the result of these experiments, which have all the accuracy of a chemical operation performed in the laboratory, and all the beauty of the most perfect injection.

"We are not, therefore, surprised that divers pathological cases, hitherto imperfectly understood, should come to confirm the views of M. Bernard, by proving that, in diseases of the pancreas, fatty matters have been observed to pass unchanged in the dejections.

"The committee cannot hesitate to conclude that the author has perfectly demonstrated his physiological propositions; that he has completed the general characters of the theory of digestion, and that he has made known the mode of formation of the fatty matter of the chyle, and the manner of the digestion of the fatty matters."

The Kidneys.—Their office is, to secrete from the blood the useless or excrementitious fluids in the form of urine. When the skin is obstructed, the secretion is augmented, and profuse perspiration lessens it. From a cavity in the centre of each kidney a canal or tube proceeds, by which the urine is conveyed into the bladder. These tubes are named *ureters.* As the ureters enter the bladder, they pass forward, a short distance between its coats; which effectually prevents the urine from taking a retrograde course. The urine is expelled by the muscular power which the bladder possesses of contracting upon its contents.

RESPIRATION AND STRUCTURE OF THE LUNGS.

THE organs of respiration are the larynx, the trachea, or windpipe, bronchia, and the lungs.

The air is expelled from the lungs principally by the action of the muscles of respiration; and when these relax, the lungs expand by virtue of their own elasticity. This may be exemplified by means of a sponge, which may be compressed into a small compass by the hand, but, upon opening the hand, the sponge returns to its natural size, and all its cavities become filled with air. The purification of the blood in the lungs is of vital importance, and indispensably necessary to the due performance of all the functions; for if they be in a diseased state, — either tuberculous, or having adhesions to the pleura, their function will be impaired; the blood will appear black; loaded with carbon; and the phlebotomizer will have the very best (worst) excuse for taking away a few quarts with a view of purifying the remainder! The trachea, or windpipe, after dividing into smaller branches, called *bronchia*, again subdivides into innumerable other branches, the extremities of which are composed of an infinite number of small cells, which, with the ramifications of veins, arteries, nerves, and connecting membranes, make up the whole mass or substance of the lungs. The internal surface of the windpipe, bronchea, and air-cells, is lined with a delicate membrane, highly organized with blood-vessels, &c. The whole is invested with a thin, transparent membrane — a continuation of that lining the chest, named *pleura*. It also covers the diaphragm, and, by a duplication of its folds, forms a separation between the lobes of the lungs.

CIRCULATION OF THE BLOOD.

THE blood contains the elements for building up, supplying the waste of, and nourishing the whole animal economy. On making an examination of the blood with a microscope, it is found full of little red globules, which vary in their size and shape in different animals, and are more numerous in the warm than in the cold-blooded. Probably this arises from the fact that the latter absorb less oxygen than the former. When blood stands for a time after being drawn, it separates into two parts. One is called *serum*. and resembles the white of an

THE HEART VIEWED EXTERNALLY.

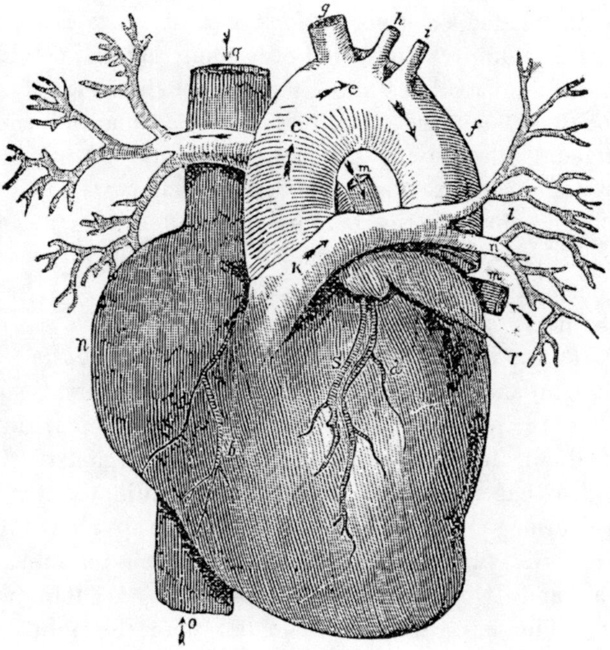

a, the left ventricle; *b*, the right ventricle; *c*, *e*, *f*, the aorta; *g*, *h*, *i*, the carotid and other arteries springing from the aorta; *k*, the pulmonary artery; *l*, branches of the pulmonary artery in the lungs; *m*, *m*, the pulmonary veins emptying into the left auricle; *n*, the right auricle; *o*, the ascending vena cava; *q*, the descending vena cava; *r*, the left auricle; *s*, the coronary vein and artery. (See ***Circulation of the Blood***, on the opposite page.)

egg; the other is the clot, or crassamentum, and form. .ed coagulum, or jelly-like substance. This is accompanied by whitish tough threads, called *fibrine*.

When blood has been drawn from an animal, and it assumes a cupped or hollow form, if serum, or buffy coat, remains on its surface, it denotes an impoverished state; but if the whole, when coagulated, be of one uniform mass, it indicates a healthy state of that fluid. The blood of a young animal, provided it be in health, coagulates into a firm mass, while that of an old or debilitated one is generally less dense, and more easily separated. The power that propels the blood through the different blood-vessels is a mechanico-vital power, and is accomplished through the involuntary contractions and relaxations of the heart; from certain parts of which arteries arise, in other parts veins terminate. (See Plate.)

The heart is invested with a strong membranous sac, called *pericardium*, which adheres to the tendinous centre of the diaphragm, and to the great vessels at its superior portion. The heart is lubricated by a serous fluid, secreted within the pericardium, for the purpose of guarding against friction. When an excess of fluid accumulates within the sac, it is termed dropsy of the heart. The heart is divided into four cavities, viz., two auricles, named from their resemblance to an ear, and two ventricles, (as seen at *a*, *b*,) forming the body. The left ventricle is smaller than the right, yet its walls are much thicker and stronger than those of the latter: it is from this part that the large trunk of the arteries proceed, called the *great aorta*. The right cavity, or ventricle, is the receptacle for blood returned by the venous structure after having gone the rounds of the circulation; the veins terminating, as they approach the heart, in a single vessel, called *vena cava*, (see plate, *o*, *q*, ascending and descending portion.) The auricle on the left side of the heart receives the blood that has been distributed through the lungs for purification. Where the veins terminate in auricles, there are valves placed, to prevent the blood from returning. For example, the blood proceeds out of the heart along the aorta; the valve opens upwards; the blood also moves upwards, and raises the valve and passes through; the pressure from above effectually closes the passage. The valves of the heart are composed of elastic cartilage, which admits of free motion. They sometimes however, become ossified. The heart and its appendages are, like other parts of the system, subject to various diseases, which are frequently very little understood, yet often fatal. Now, the blood, having passed through the veins and vena cava, flows into the right auricle; and this, when distended, contracts, and forces its contents into the right ventricle, which, contracting in its turn, propels the blood into the pulmonary arteries, whose numerous ramifications bring it in contact with the air-cells of the lungs. It then, being deprived of its carbon, assumes a crimson color. Having passed through its proper vessels, it accumulates in the left auricle. This also contracts, and forces the blood through a valve into the left ventricle. This ventricle then contracts in its turn, and the blood passes through another valve into the great aorta, to go the round of the circulation and return in the manner just described.

Many interesting experiments have been made to estimate the quantity of blood in an animal. "The weight of a dog," says Mr. Percival, "being ascertained to be seventy-nine pounds, a puncture was made with the lancet into the jugular vein, from which the blood was collected. The vein having ceased to bleed, the carotid artery of the same side was divided, but no blood came from it; in a few seconds afterwards, the animal was dead. The weight of the carcass was now found to be seventy-three and a half pounds; consequently it had sustained a loss of five and a half pounds — precisely the measure of the blood drawn. It appears from this experiment, that an animal will lose about one fifteenth part of its weight of blood before it dies; though a less quantity may so far debilitate the vital powers, as to be, though less suddenly, equally fatal. In the human subject, the quantity of blood has been computed at about one eighth part of the weight of the body; and as such an opinion has been broached from the results of experiments on quadrupeds, we may fairly take that to be about the proportion of it in the horse; so that if we estimate the weight of a horse to be thirteen hundred and forty-four pounds, the whole quantity of blood will amount to eighty-four quarts, or one hundred and sixty-eight pounds; of which about forty-five quarts, or ninety pounds, will commonly flow from the jugular vein prior to death; though the loss of a much less quantity will deprive the animal of life.

REMARKS ON BLOOD-LETTING.

The author has been, for several years, engaged in a warfare against the use of the lancet in the treatment of the various diseases of animals. When this warfare was first commenced, the prospect was poor indeed. The lancet was the great anti-phlogistic of the allopathic school; it had powerful, talented, and uncompromising advocates, who had been accustomed to resort to it on all occasions, from the early settlement of America up to that period. The great mass had followed in the footsteps of their predecessors, supposing them to be infallible. Men and animals were bled; rivers of blood have been drawn from their systems; yet they often got well, and men looked upon the lancet as one of the blessings of the age, when, in fact, it is the greatest curse that ever afflicted this country: it has produced greater losses to owners of domestic animals than did ever pestilence or disease. A few philanthropic practitioners have, from time to time, in other countries, as well as in this, labored during their life, and on their death-bed, to convince the world of the destructive tendency of blood-letting in human practice; but none that we know of ever had the moral courage to wage a general warfare against the practice in the veterinary department, until we commenced it. We have met with great success, and have given the blood-letting gentry who practise it at the present day ("just to please their employers or to make out a case") a partial quietus: in a few more years, unless they abandon their false theories, their occupation, notwithstanding their pretensions to cure *secundum artem*, will, like Othello's, be "gone." But we are not writing for doctors. Our business is with the farmers — the lords of creation. The former are mere lords of pukes and purges; they, like the farmers, have the materials, however, to mould themselves into men of common sense; but the fact is, they are hide-bound; they want a national sweat, to rid their systems, especially their upper works, of the theories of Sydenham and Paracelsus, which have shipwrecked many thousands of the medical profession. They shut their eyes to the results of medical reform, and cling, with all their soul, and with all their might, worthy a better cause, to a system that "always was false."

Lord Byron, like many other learned men, was well acquainted with the impotency of the healing art, and held the lancet in utter abhorrence: when beset, day and night, to be bled, the bard, in an angry tone, exclaimed, "You are, I see, a d——d set of butchers; take away as much blood as you like." "We seized the opportunity," says Dr. Milligan, "and drew twenty ounces; yet the relief did not correspond to the hopes we had formed." On the 17th, the bleeding was twice repeated, dangerous symptoms still increasing, and on the 19th he expired, just about bled to death. Washington, a man whose name is dear to every American, died from the effects of an evil system of medication. He was attacked with croup: his physician bled him, and gave him calomel and antimony. The next day, physicians were called in, (to share the responsibility of the butchery,) and he was subjected to two more copious bleedings: in all he lost ninety ounces of blood. Which of our readers, at the present day, would submit to such unwarrantable barbarity? We just said we were not writing for doctors; yet we find ourselves off the track in thus administering a small dose, as a sample of "*good and efficient treatment.*"

In reference to the success attending our labors in veterinary reform, we do not claim the whole credit: much of it is due to the intelligence of the American farmers, in appreciating the value and importance of a safer and a more effectual system of medication; such a system as we advocate They have witnessed the results attending the practice of cattle doctors generally, and they have seen the results of our sanative system of medication, and a great majority in Massachusetts have decided in favor of the latter. We have demonstrated to the satisfaction of our patrons, and we are ready and willing to repeat our experiments on diseased animals for the satisfaction of others, in showing that we can restore an animal, when suffering under acute attacks of disease, in a few hours, when, by the popular method, it takes weeks and months, if indeed they ever recover from the effects of the destructive agents used.

We are told that "horses and cattle are bled and get well immediately." This may apply to some cases; but, in very many instances, the animals are sent for a few weeks to "Dr. Green,"* to put them in the same condition they were at the time of bleeding. But suppose that some animals do get well after bleeding; is it thus proved that more would not get well if no blood were drawn from any? A cow may fall down, and, in so doing, lacerate her muscles, blood-vessels, &c., and lose a large quantity of blood. She may get well, in spite of the violence and loss of blood. So we say of blood-letting, if the abstraction of a certain number of gallons of blood will kill a strong animal, then the abstraction of a small quantity must injure it proportionately.

There is in the animal economy a power, called the vital principle, which always operates in favor of health. If the provocation be gentle, and does not seriously derange the machinery, then this power may overcome both it and any disease the animal may at the time labor under. For example, a horse falls down in the street, perhaps laboring under a

* A piece of pasture land.

temporary congestion of the brain: now, if he were let alone until nature has restored an equilibrium of the circulating fluid and nervous action, he would soon get up and proceed on his way, as many thousands do when a knife or lancet is not to be had. But, unfortunately, people are too hasty. The moment a beast has fallen, they are bound to have him on his perpendiculars in double quick time. The teamster cannot wait for nature; she is "too slow a coach" for him. He tries what virtue there is in the whip; this failing, he obtains a knife, if one is to be had, and "*starts the blood.*" By this time, nature, about resuming her empire, causes the horse to show signs of returning animation, and the credit is awarded to the blood-starter. Animals are often bled when diseased, and the prominent symptoms that previously marked the character of the malady disappear, or give place to symptoms of another order, less evident, and men have supposed that a cure is effected, when, in fact, they have just sown the seeds of a future disease. We are not bound to prove, in every case, how an animal gets well after two or three repeated bleedings. It is enough for us to prove that this operation always tends to death, which can easily be produced by opening the carotid artery of an animal.

Permit us, dear reader, at this stage of our article, to observe, that "confession is good for the soul." We mean to put it in practice. So here goes. We plead guilty to bleeding, blistering, calomelizing, narcotizing, antimonializing, a great number of patients of the human kind. We did it in our verdant days, because it was so scientific and popular, and because we had been taught to reverence the stereotyped practice of the allopathists. We have, however, done penance, and sought forgiveness; and through the aid of a few men, devoted to medical reform, we have been washed in the regenerating waters flowing through the vineyard of reason and experience, and now advocate and observe the self-regulating powers of the laws of life. On the other hand, we are free from the charge of bleeding or poisoning domestic animals, and can say, with a clear conscience, that we have never drawn a drop of blood from a four-footed creature, (except in surgical operations, when it could not be avoided;) neither will we, under any circumstances, resort to the lancet; for we are convinced that blood-letting is a powerful depressor of the vital powers.

Blood is the fuel that keeps the lamp of life burning; if the fuel be withdrawn, the light is extinguished.

Professor Lobstein says, "So far from blood-letting being beneficial, it is productive of the most serious consequences — a cruel practice, and a scourge to humanity. How many thousands are sent by it to an untimely grave! Without blood there is no heat, no motion in the body."

Dr. Reid says, "If the employment of the lancet was abolished altogether, it would perhaps save annually a greater number of lives than pestilence ever destroyed."

The fact of blood-letting having been practised by horse and cattle doctors from time immemorial is certainly not a clear proof of its utility, nor is it a sufficient recommendation that it may be practised with safety. During my professional career, the preconceived theories have commanded a due share of consideration; and, when weighed in the scale of uninfluenced experience, they never failed of falling short. If we grant that any deviation from the healthy state denotes debility of one or more functions, then whatever has a tendency to debilitate further cannot restore the animal to health. The following case will serve to illustrate our position: "A horse was brought to be bled, merely because he had been accustomed to it at that season of the year. I did not examine him minutely; but as the groom stated there was nothing amiss with him, I directed a moderate quantity of blood to be drawn. About five pints were taken off; and while the operator was pinning up the wound, the horse fell. He appeared to suffer much pain, and had considerable difficulty of breathing. In this state he remained twelve hours, and then died. Judging from the appearances at the post mortem examination, it is probable that a loss of a moderate quantity of blood caused a fatal interruption of the functions of the heart."

It is strange that such cases as these do not open men's eyes, and compel them to acknowledge that there is something wrong in the medical world. Such cases as these furnish us with unanswerable arguments against blood-letting; for as the blood, which is the natural stimulus of, and gives strength to, the organs, is withdrawn, its abstraction leaves all those organs less capable of self-defence.

Horse and cattle doctors have recommended bleeding when animals have been fed too liberally, or if their systems abound in morbific matter. Now, the most sensible course would be, provided the animal had been overfed, to reduce the quantity of food, or, in other words, remove the cause. If the secretions are vitiated, or in a morbid state, then regulate them by the means laid down in this work. For we cannot purify a well of water by abstracting a few buckets; neither can we purify the whole mass of blood by taking away a few quarts; for that which is left will still be impure. If the different parts had between them partitions impervious to fluids, then there would be some sense in drawing out of the vessels overfilled; but unfortunately, if you draw from one, you draw from all the rest.

In every disease wherein bleeding has been used, complete recovery has been protracted, and the animal manifests the debility by swelled legs and other unmistakable evidences. In some cases, however, the ill effects of the loss of blood, unless excessive, are not always immediately perceived; yet such animals, in after years, are subject to staggers, and diseases of the lungs, pleura, and peritoneum.

Dr. Beach says, "The blood is properly called the *vital fluid*, and the life of a person is said to be in the blood.* We know that just in proportion to the loss of this substance are our vigor and strength taken from us. When taken from the system by accident or the lancet, it is succeeded by great prostration of strength, and a derangement of all the functions

* Then the life of an animal is also in the blood; and the same evil consequences follow its abstraction.

of the body. These effects are invariably, in a greater or less degree, consequent on bleeding. Is it not, then, reasonable to suppose, that what will debilitate the strongest constitution in a state of health, will be attended with most serious evils when applied to a person laboring under any malady? Is it not like throwing spirits on a fire to extinguish it?

"Bleeding is resorted to in all inflammatory complaints; but did practitioners know the nature and design of inflammation, their treatment would be different. In fever it is produced by an increased action of the heart and arteries, to expel acrid and noxious humors, and should be promoted until the irritating matter is dislodged from the system. This should be effected, in general, by opening the outlets of the body, inducing perspiration; to produce which a preternatural degree of heat or inflammation must be excited by internal remedies. Fever is nothing more or less than a wholesome and salutary effort of nature to throw off some morbific matter; and, therefore, every means to lessen this indication proves injurious. Bleeding, in consequence of the debility it produces, prevents such indication from being fulfilled."

The inveterate phlebotomizers recommend and practise bleeding when "*the animal has too much blood.*" There may be at times too much blood, and at others too little; but suppose there is,—has any body found out any better method of reducing what they please to term an excess, than that of regular exercise in the open air, combined with a less quantity of fodder than usual? Or has any body found out any method of making good healthy blood, other than the slow process of nature, as exhibited in the results of digestion, secretion, circulation, and nutrition? Have they discovered any artificial means of restoring the blood to its healthful quantity when it is deficient? Have they found any means of purifying the blood, save the healthful operations of nature's secreting and excreting laboratory? Finally, have they found any safety-valve or outlet for the reduction of this excess other than the excrementitious vessels? And if they have, are they better able to adjust the pressure on that valve than

He who made the whole machinery, and knows the relative strength of all its parts? In an article on blood-letting, found in the Farmer's Cyclopædia, the author says, "In summer, bleeding is often necessary to prevent fevers." Now, it is evident that nature's preventives are air, exercise, food, water, and sleep. Attention to the rules laid down in this work, under the heads of *Watering*, *Feeding*, &c., will be more satisfactory and less dangerous than that recommended by the Cyclopædia. If the directions given in the latter were fully carried out, the stock of our farms would be swept away as by the blast of a tornado. Such a barbarous system would entail universal misery and degeneracy on all classes of live stock; and we might then exclaim, "They are living, yet half dead — victims to an inconsistent system of medication!" But thanks to a discerning public, they just begin to see the absurdity and wickedness of draining the system of the living principles. Veterinary reform has germinated in the New England States, and, in spite of all opposition, has struck its roots deep into the minds of a class of men who have the means and power to send forth its healing branches, and apply them to their own interest and the welfare of their stock.

The same author continues: "Some farriers bleed horses three or four times a year." We hope the farmers have too much good sense to follow the wicked example of the former. Frequent bleeding is an indirect mode of butchery — killing by inches; for it gives to the blood-vessels the power to contract and adapt themselves to the measure of blood that remains. It impoverishes the blood, and leads to hydrothorax, (accumulation of water in the chest,) and materially shortens life. Mackintosh says, "Some are bled who cannot bear it, and others who do not require it; and the result is death." The conservative power of life always operates in favor of health, and resists the encroachments upon her province with all her might, and often recovers the dominion; but by frequent bleedings, she is exhausted, and, on taking a little more blood than usual, the animal drops down and dies; and the owner attributes to disease what, in fact, is the result of bad treatment.

"Patients who recover after general and copious bleedings have been employed, may attribute their recovery to the strength of their constitution.

"If you should ask a modern *Sangrado* what was most necessary in the treatment of disease, doubtless he would reply, 'Bleeding.'"

"Our modern pathologists, surgeons and others, think bleeding the *factotum* in all maladies; it is the *ne plus ultra*, when drawn in large quantities. Blood-letting, say these authors, is not only the most powerful and important, but the most generally used, of all our remedies. Scarcely a case of acute, or, indeed, of chronic, disease occurs in which it does not become necessary to consider the propriety of having recourse to the lancet." (? ?) To what extent blood-letting is carried, in our modern age, may be learned by reading Youatt and others, who recommend it "when animals rub themselves, and the hair falls off; when the eyes appear dull and languid, red or inflamed; in all inflammatory complaints, as of the brain, lungs, kidneys, bowels, womb, bladder, and joints; in all bruises, hurts, wounds, and all other accidents; in cold, catarrh, paralysis, and locked-jaw." Yet, strange to say, one of these authors qualifies his recommendations as follows: "No man, however wise, can tell exactly how much blood ought to be taken in a given case." Now, it is well known that the draining of blood from a vein, though it diminishes the vital resistance, and lessens the volume of fluids, does not mend the matter; for it thus gives to cold and atmospheric agents the ascendant influence. A collapse takes place, the secretions become impaired, the animal refuses its food, "looks dumpish," &c.

We might continue this article to an indefinite length; but as we shall, in the following pages, have occasion to refer to the use of the lancet as a destructive agent, we conclude it with the following remarks of an English physician: "Our most valuable remedies against inflammation are but ill adapted for curing that state of disease. They do not act directly on the diseased part; the action is only indirect; therefore it is imperfect. Bleeding, the best of any of these remedies, is in this predicament."

EFFORTS OF NATURE TO REMOVE DISEASE.

"Nature is ever busy, by the silent operations of her own forces, in curing disease." — *Dixon.*

WHENEVER any irritating substance comes in contact with sensitive surfaces, nature, or the *vis medicatrix naturæ*, goes immediately to work to remove the offending cause: for example, should any substance lodge on the mucous surface, within the nostril, although it be imperceptible, as often happens when the hay is musty, it abounds in particles whose specific gravity enables them to float in atmospheric air; they are then inhaled in the act of respiration, and nature, in order to wash off the offending matter, sends a quantity of fluid to the part. The same process may be observed when a small piece of hay, or other foreign matter, shall have fallen into the eye: the tears then flow in great abundance, to prevent that delicate organ being injured. "When a blister is applied to the surface, it first excites a genial warmth, with inflammation of the skin; and nature, distressed, goes instantly to work, separates the cuticle to form a bag, interposes serum between the nerves and the offensive matter, then prepares another cuticle, that, when the former, with the adhering substance, shall fall off, the nervous papillæ may be again provided with a covering.

"The same reasoning will apply to the operation of emetics and cathartics; for not only is the peristaltic motion either greatly quickened or inverted, according to the urgency of the distress, but both the mucous glands and the exhalent arteries pour forth their fluids in abundance to wash away the offending matter, which at one time acts chemically, at others mechanically."

If a horse, or an ox, be wounded in the foot with a nail

and a portion of it is broken off and remains in the wound, inflammation sets in, producing suppuration, and the nail is discharged.

A few days ago, we were called to see a horse, said to have a swelling on the *tarsus*, (hock.) On an examination, it proved to be an abscess, well developed; the matter could be distinctly felt at the most prominent part. We should certainly have been justified (at least in the eyes of the medical world; and then it would have looked so "doctor-like"!) in displaying a case of instruments and opening the tumor. If ulceration, gangrene, &c., set in, and the horse ultimately became lame, no blame could be attached to us, because the practice is *scientific!* — recognized by the schools as good and efficient treatment. What was to be done? Why, it was evident that we could not do better than to aid nature. A relaxing, anti-spasmodic poultice was confined to the parts, and in six hours after, the sac discharged its contents, and with it a piece of splinter two inches in length. The pain immediately ceased, and the animal is now free from lameness. We here see the design of nature: the consequent inflammation was to produce suppuration, and make an outlet for the splinter.

Professor Kost says, "The laws of all organic life are remarkably peculiar; they possess, in an eminent degree, the power of self-regulation. When interrupted, disease, indeed, supervenes; but unless the circumstances are particularly unfavorable, the physiological state will soon be restored. All observation most clearly corroborates this fact. The healing of wounds, restoration of fractured bones, expulsion of obtruded substances, and particularly the manner in which extravasated matter or pus is removed from internal organs, as in case of abscess in the liver, in which exit may be gained by ulceration through the parietes, or by an adhesion to and ulceration into the intestines, or even by the adhesions to the diaphragm and lungs, in such a manner as, by ulceration into the bronchia, a passage may be gained, and the pus thus removed by expectoration, — all evince a most singular conservative power. What is most remarkable in cases like the latter, is, that the adhesions are so formed as to prevent the escape of the pus into the peritoneal sac, which accident must inevitably prove fatal.

"Some very interesting experiments have been performed to test the restorative power of the different tissues of the animal body. If a portion of the intestines of a dog be taken out, and tied, so as to obstruct completely the passage, it will be found that the adjacent portions of the intestine will reunite, the ligature will separate into the canal and be discharged, and the gut will heal up so as to preserve its normal continuity, and the animal, in a fortnight, will have recovered entirely from the effects of this fearful operation.

"When noxious or poisonous substances are thrown into any of the cavities of the body from which their escape is impracticable, a cyst will often form around them, and they thus become isolated from absorption and the circulation, so as to prevent their doing harm.

"The less remarkable instances of this character are of more common occurrence; and the self-regulating power of the laws of life, alias *vis conservatrix naturæ*, is so universally known and depended on, that it is rare, indeed, that indisposed persons take medicine, until they have first waited at least a little, to see what nature would do for them; and they are seldom disappointed, as it may perhaps be safely asserted, that nine tenths of all the attacks of disease (taking the slight indispositions; for such are most of them, as they are checked before they become severe) are warded off by the vital force, unassisted. Such, then, are the facts deduced from observing the operations of nature in disease *unassisted.*"

Dr. Beach says, "We are well aware, from what passes in the system daily, that the Author of nature has wisely provided a principle which is calculated to remove disease. It is very observable in fevers. No sooner is noxious or morbid matter retained in the system, than there is an increased action of the heart and arteries, to eliminate the existing cause from the skin; or it may pass off by other outlets established for that purpose. With what propriety, then, can this provision of nature be denied, as it is by some? A noted professor in Philadelphia or Baltimore ridicules this power in the constitution; he says to his class, 'Kick nature out of doors.' It was this man, or a brother professor, who exclaimed to his class, 'Give me mercury in one hand and the lancet in the other, and I am prepared to cope with disease in every shape and form.' I have not time to stop here, and comment upon such palpable and dangerous doctrine. I have only to say, let the medical historian record this sentiment, maintained in the highest medical universities in America in the nineteenth century. I am pleased, however, to observe, that all physicians do not coincide with such views."

PROVERBS OF THE VETERINARY REFORMERS.

The merciful man is merciful to his domestic animals.

"Avoid blood-letting and poisons, for they are powerful depressors of the vital energies. There are two medical *fulcra* — reason and experience. Experience precedes, reason follows; hence, reasoning not founded on experience avails nothing. He who cures by simples need not seek for compounds." — *Villanov.*

"The physician *destitute of a knowledge of plants* can never properly judge of the power of a plant." — *Whitlaw.*

"The vegetable kingdom is the most noble in medicines." — *Ibid.*

Innocent medicines, which approach as near to food as possible, preserve health, while chemical compounds destroy it. Heroic medicines (such are antimony, copper, corrosive sublimate, lead, opium, hellebore, arsenic, belladonna) are like the sword in the hands of a madman.

"Nature unassisted by art sometimes effects miracles." — *Whitlaw.*

"It is the part of a wise physician to decline prescribing in a lost case." — *Ibid.* Whenever there is free, full circulation of blood, there is animal heat. If the heat of a part becomes deficient, the circulation is correspondingly diminished. As soon as voluntary motion in a part ceases, so soon the circulation becomes enfeebled; and if continued, the part will wither and waste away.

The strength and health of an animal depend on a due share of exercise, pure air, and suitable food. Deprive an animal of these, and he will cease to exist. We believe in the great doctrine that the duty of the physician is to aid nature in protecting herself in the enjoyment of health, by proper attention to breeding, rearing, ventilation, and proper farm and stable management.

"The tinsel glitter of fine-spun theory, or favorite hypothesis, which prevails wherever allopathy hath been taught, so dazzles, flatters, and charms human vanity and folly, that, so far from contributing to the certain and speedy cure of diseases, it hath, in every age, proved the bane and disgrace of the healing art." — *Graham*, p. 15.

"Those physicians generally become the most distinguished who soonest emancipate themselves from the tyranny of the schools of physic." — *Rush.*

"Availing ourselves of the privileges we possess, and animated by the noblest impulses, let us cordially coöperate to give to medicine a new direction, and attempt those great improvements which it imperiously demands." — *Ther.*, vol. i. p. 51.

"It has been proved by allopathists themselves, that 'a physician should be nature's servant;' that 'bleeding tends directly to subdue nature's efforts;' that 'all poisons suddenly and rapidly destroy a great proportion of the vitality of the system;' that whatever be the quantity, use, or manner of application, all the influence they inherently possess is injurious, and that they are not fatal in every instance of their use only because nature overpowers them." — *Curtis.*

AN INQUIRY CONCERNING THE SOULS OF BRUTES.

"Are these then made in vain? Is man alone,
Of all the marvels of creative love,
Blest with a scintillation of His essence —
The heavenly spark of reasonable soul?
And hath not yon sagacious dog, that finds
A meaning in the shepherd's idiot face;
Or the huge elephant, that lends his strength
To drag the stranded galley to the shore,
And strives with emulative pride t' excel
The mindless crowd of slaves that toil beside him;
Or the young generous war-horse, when he sniffs
The distant field of blood, and quick and shrill
Neighing for joy, instils a desperate courage
Into the veteran trooper's quailing heart, —
Have they not all an evidence of soul,
(Of soul, the proper attribute of man,)
The same in kind, though meaner in degree?
Why should not that which hath been — be forever?
And death, O, can it be annihilation?
No, — though the stolid atheist fondly clings
To that last hope, how kindred to despair!
No, — 'tis the struggling spirit's hour of joy,
The glad emancipation of the soul,
The moment when the cumbrous fetters drop,
And the bright spirit wings its way to heaven!

"To say that God annihilated aught,
Were to declare that in an unwise hour
He planned and made somewhat superfluous.
Why should not the mysterious life that dwells
In reptiles as in man, and shows itself
In memory, gratitude, love, hate, and pride,
Still energize, and be, though death may crush
Yon frugal ant or thoughtless butterfly,
Or, with the simoom's pestilential gale
Strike down the patient camel in the desert?

"There is one chain of intellectual soul,

In many links and various grades, throughout
The scale of nature; from the climax bright,
The first great Cause of all, Spirit supreme,
Incomprehensible, and unconfined,
To high archangels blazing near the throne,
Seraphim, cherubim, virtues, aids, and powers,
All capable of perfection in their kind; —
To man, as holy from his Maker's hand
He stood in possible excellence complete,
(Man, who is destined now to brighter glories, —
As nearer to the present God, in One
His Lord and Substitute, — than angels reach;)
Then man has fallen, with every varied shade
Of character and capability,
From him who reads his title to the skies,
Or grasps, with giant-mind, all nature's wonders,
Down to the monster-shaped, inhuman form,
Murderer, slavering fool, or blood-stained savage:
Then to the prudent elephant, the dog
Half-humanized, the docile Arab horse,
The social beaver, and contriving fox,
The parrot, quick in pertinent reply,
The kind-affectioned seal, and patriot bee,
The merchant-storing ant, and wintering swallow
With all those other palpable emanations
And energies of one Eternal Mind
Pervading and instructing all that live,
Down to the sentient grass and shrinking clay
In truth, I see not why the breath of life,
Thus omnipresent, and upholding all,
Should not return to Him and be immortal.
(I dare not say the same,) in some glad state
Originally destined for creation,
As well from brutish bodies, as from man.
The uncertain glimmer of analogy
Suggests the thought, and reason's shrewder guess;
Yet revelation whispers nought but this, —
'Our Father careth when a sparrow dies,
And that 'the spirit of a brute descends,'
As to some secret and preserving Hades.

"But for some better life, in what strange sort
Were justice, mixed with mercy, dealt to these?
Innocent slaves of sordid, guilty man,
Poor unthanked drudges, toiling to his will,
Pampered in youth, and haply starved in age.
Obedient, faithful, gentle, though the spur,
Wantonly cruel, or unsparing thong,
Weal your galled hides, or your strained sinews crack
Beneath the crushing load, — what recompense
Can He who gave you being render you,
If in the rank, full harvest of your griefs
Ye sink annihilated, to the shame
Of government unequal? — In that day
When crime is sentenced, shall the cruel heart
Boast uncondemned, because no tortured brute
Stands there accusing? Shall the embodied deeds
Of man not follow him, nor the rescued fly
Bear its kind witness to the saving hand?
Shall the mild Brahmin stand in equal sin
Regarding nature's menials, with the wretch
Who flays the moaning Abyssinian ox,
Or roasts the living bird, or flogs to death
The famishing pointer? — and must these again,
These poor, unguilty, uncomplaining victims,
Have no reward for life with its sharp pains? —
They have my suffrage: Nineveh was spared,
Though Jonah prophesied its doom, for sake
Of sixscore thousand infants, and 'much cattle;'
And space is wide enough for every grain
Of the broad sands that curb our swelling seas,
Each separate in its sphere to stand apart
As far as sun from sun; there lacks not room,
Nor time, nor care, where all is infinite." — *Tupper*

THE REFORMED PRACTICE.

SYNOPTICAL VIEW OF THE PROMINENT SYSTEMS OF MEDICINE.

Some of our readers, especially the non-medical, may desire to know what the following remarks, which appear to apply generally to the human family, have to do with cattle doctoring. We answer them in the language of Professor Percival. "The object of the veterinary art is not only congenial with human medicine, but the very same paths which lead to a knowledge of the diseases of man, lead also to a knowledge of those of brutes. An accurate examination of the interior parts of their bodies; a studious survey of the arrangement, structure, use, connection, and relation of these parts, and of the laws by which they act; as also of the nature and properties of the various food and other agents which the earth so liberally provides for their support and cure, — these form, in a great measure, the sound and sure foundation of all medical science, whatever living individual animal be the subject of our consideration. Whether we prescribe for a man, horse, dog, or cat, the laws of the animal economy are the same; and one system, and that based upon established facts, is to guide our practice in all.

"The theory of medicine in the human subject is the theory of medicine in the brute; it is the application of that theory — the practice alone — that is different.

"We might as well, in reference to the principles of each, attempt to separate surgery from medicine, as insist that either of these arts, in theory, is essentially different from the veterinary: every day's experience serves to confirm this our belief, and in showing us how often the diseases of animals arise from the same causes as those of a man, exhibit the same indications, and require a similar method of cure.

"The science of medicine, like others, consists of a collection of facts of a common and not a specific character.

These, therefore, admit of arrangement into different systems, according to the notions of theorists, and the various species of philosophy, brought to bear on the subject.

"The first regular system was founded by Hippocrates, about three hundred and eighty years before Christ. It was founded upon *theory*, and comprised the doctrines of the ancient dogmatic school. Its pathology rested upon a supposed change of the humors of the body, particularly the blood and bile; and here are the first elements of the '*humoral pathology*.' Its remedial intentions were founded upon the existence of the '*vis conservatrix*' *et* '*medicatrix naturæ;*' and, although often maintaining direct antipathic principles of action, it rested mainly on physo-dynamic influence for the accomplishment of its therapeutic purposes.

"About two hundred and ninety years before Christ, Philinus of Cos introduced the ancient *Empiric System*, which was founded upon *experience* and *observation*. About one hundred years before the Christian era, the *Methodic System* was introduced by Asclepiades of Bithynia. This system was got up with an avowed opposition to that of Hippocrates, which was called 'a study of death.' Themison of Laodicea, pupil of Asclepiades, gives an exposition of the fundamental principles of the methodic system; and it seems that all physiological and pathological action was considered to be dependent upon the *strictum* and *laxum* of the organic pores, or increased and decreased secretion, and that all medicines act only on two principles, *i. e.*, by inducing contraction and relaxation, or an increase and decrease of the secretions.

"It would seem that, in the first century of the Christian era, the methodic system was divided into various subordinate ones — the *Pneumatic*, *Episynthetic*, and *Eclectic*. The pneumatic system, which was the most popular of the fragments of the methodic, was most indebted to Athenæus of Attalia for its successful introduction. This system contemplated the doctrine of the Stoics, which recognized the existence of a spirit governing and directing every thing, and which, when offended, would produce disease; hence the name *pneumatic.* The indications of cure were more *moral* than *physical.* Fire, air, water, &c., were not considered elements, but their properties — heat, cold, dryness, moisture, &c. — were alone entitled to the name.

"In the second century, the *Galenic System* was founded by Claudius Galenus. This might, indeed, only be considered the revival of the dogmatic or Hippocratean system. Galen professed to have selected what he found valuable from all the prevailing systems, and has embraced the elements and ruling spirit of the pneumatic school. Thus he explained the operation of medicines by reference to their elementary qualities, — that is, heat, cold, dryness, and moisture, — of each of which he admitted four degrees. But he was governed by a prevailing partiality for the system of Hippocrates, which, he states, was either misunderstood or misrepresented by all theorists, ever since the establishment of the empiric and methodic schools. He devoted most of his time to commenting upon and embellishing it, and thus again established a system, founded on reason, observation, and sound induction, which maintained its character, without a rival, for more than one thousand five hundred years.

"Near the middle of the sixteenth century, Paracelsus introduced the *Chemical System.* This was strongly opposed by Bellonius and Riverius, who maintained the doctrine of Hippocrates and Galen. But the presumptuous Paracelsus burned, 'in solemn state,' the works of the ancients; and being succeeded by the indefatigable Van Helmont, the whole science of medicine was overwhelmed by the mysticism of the alchemical doctrines and languages. The chemical theory, in the main, rejects the influence, or even the existence, of the *vis medicatrix naturæ*, and explains all physiological, pathological, and therapeutic operations upon abstract chemical laws. Thus chemical or inorganic agents, and many of the most virulent poisons, as arsenic, mercury, antimony, &c., were placed among the most prominent remedies.

"Soon after the introduction of the chemical system, medical science, if we make one exception, became less eccentric, but much less marked for the permanency of its systems. Boerhaave ingeniously blended most of the prominent doctrines of the Galenic and chemical systems; and by an application of several of the newly-developed natural sciences, especially mathematics and natural philosophy, he led his successors into a more even path and fixed method of investigation; for no more do we find any abstract physical laws the sole basis of a system. But these were the highest honors allowed Boerhaave; his particular system was soon subverted by Stahl, who proved the supreme superintendence of an immaterial, vital principle, corresponding to that pointed out by Hippocrates. To this he ascribes intelligence, if not moral attributes. Hoffman led Cullen into the path that brought him into the fruitful field of the *nervous pathology* and solidism, which, with a modification of Stahl's ruling *immaterial essence*, formed the groundwork of his admired system.

"If, now, we except the eccentricities of Brown, comprising his system, founded on the *sthenic* and *asthenic* diathesis, we find little interruption to the general prevalence of the Cullenian system, till nearly the present juncture. The succeeding authors, colleges, and medical societies have only modified and amplified the general theory, and regulated the practice into a comparative uniformity, which now constitutes the popular *Allopathic System.* But notwithstanding the comparatively settled state of medical science, it could not be supposed that in this remarkable age of improvement, while all other liberal sciences and arts are progressing as if prosecuted by superhuman agency, medicine should fail to undergo corresponding improvement.

"Several new systems of medicine date themselves within the last forty years, viz.: 1. The *Homœopathic*, introduced by Hahnemann, and founded upon the principle, *similia similibus curantur.* 2. The *Botanic*, established by a new class of medical philosophers, within the last twenty years. 3. The *Eclectic*, corresponding, in its essential doctrines, with the ancient eclectic system."

CREED OF THE REFORMERS.

We believe that a perfect system of medical science is that which never allows disease to exist at all; which prevents disease, instead of curing it, by means of a perfect hygienic system, proper modes of life, attention to diet, ventilation, and exercise.

We believe that the next best system is that which, after disease has made its appearance, promptly meets its development by the use of such agencies as are perfectly in harmony with the laws of life and health, and physiological in their action; such, for example, as water, air, heat and cold, friction, food, drink, and medicines that are not usually regarded as poisons, and are known to prove congenial to the animal constitution.

We have no attachment to any remedy which experience shows unsafe; but, on the contrary, we rejoice in the success of every attempt to substitute sanative for disease-creating agents, and believe that a number of the articles which are still occasionally used in the old school, will in time become obsolete, as medical science progresses.

We hold that our opposition to any course of medical treatment should be in proportion to the mischief it produces, entirely irrespective of medical theories. Hence our hostility to the lancet.

We do not profess to know more about anatomy, physiology, surgery, &c., than our allopathic brethren; but the superiority which our system claims over others is, in the main, to be found in our therapeutic agents, all of which are harmless, safe, and efficient. While they arouse the energies of nature to resist the ravages of disease, they act harmoniously with the vital principle, in the restoration of the system from a pathological to the physiological state.

TRUE PRINCIPLES.

"Our objection to the old school," says Professor Curtis, "has ever been, that they not only have no true principles to guide their practice, but they have adopted, fixed, and obstinately adhered to principles the very reverse of the true. They have resolved that, in disease, nature turns a somerset — reverses all her normal laws, and requires them to do the same. They have decreed that the best means and processes to cure the sick are those which will most speedily kill them when in health. In the face of all reason and common sense, they have adhered to this doctrine and practice for the last three centuries, and they have been constrained to confess that the destruction they have produced on human life and health has far exceeded all that has been effected by the sword, pestilence, and famine. Still they obstinately persevere. They say their science is progressive — improving; yet its progression consists in contriving new ways and means to take part of the life's blood, and poison all the balance.

"Medicine, being based on the laws of nature, is in itself an exact science; and every process of the act should be directed by those laws.

"Medicine is a demonstrative science, and all its processes should be based on fixed laws, and be governed by positive inductions. Then, and not till then, will it deserve to be ranked among the exact sciences, and contemplated as a liberal art.

"Truth is stationary; it never progresses. What was true in principle in the days of Adam is so still. To talk of progress in principle is ridiculous. Neither does a given practice progress. That which was ever intrinsically good is so still. To talk, then, of the progress in principles of medicine is absurd. We may learn the truth or error of principles, and the comparative value or worthlessness of practices; but the principles are still the same. This is our progress in knowledge, not the progress of science or art. The constant changes that have taken place in the adoption and rejection of various principles and practices have ever been an injury to the healing art. Both truth and falsehood, separately and combined, have been alternately received and rejected; and this is that progress which is made in a circle, and not in lines direct. The fault of the cultivators of medicine has been, not that they never discovered the truth nor adopted the right practice, but that they adopted wrong principles and practices as often as the right, and rejected the right as readily as the wrong. They have ever been ready to prove many, if not all things; but to cast off the bad and hold fast to the good, they seem to have had but little discrimination and power. They say truly, that the object of the healing art is to aid nature in the prevention and cure of her diseases; yet, in practice, they do violence to nature in the use of the lancet and poison."

We are told by the professors of allopathy that their medicines constitute a class of deadly poisons, (see "Pocket Pharmacopœia;") "that, when given with a scientific hand, in small doses, they cure disease." We deny their power to cure. If antimony, corrosive sublimate, &c., ever proved destructive, they always possess that power, and can never be used with any degree of assurance that they will make a sick animal well. On the other hand, we have abundant everyday evidence of their ability to make a well animal sick at any time. What difference does it make whether poisons are given with a scientific or an unscientific hand? Does it alter the tendency which all poisons possess, namely, that of rapidly depriving the system of vitality?

The veterinary science was ushered into existence by men who practised according to the doctrines of the theoretical schools. We may trace it in its infancy when, in England, in the year 1788, it was rocked in the cradle of allopathy by Sainbel, its texture varying to suit the skill of Clark, Lawrence, Field, Blaine, and Coleman; yet with all their amount of talent and wisdom, their pupils must acknowledge that the melancholy triumph of disease over its victims clearly evinces that their combined stock of knowledge is insufficient to perfect the veterinary science. Dr. J. Bell says, "Anatomy is the basis of medical skill;" yet, in another part of his work he says, "It enables the physician to GUESS *at the seat, or causes, or consequences of disease!*" This is what we propose hereafter to call the science — the science of guessing! If such is the immense mortality in England, (amounting, as Mr. Youatt states, in loss of cattle, alone, to $50,000,000,) — a country that boasts of her veterinary institutions, and embraces within her medical halo some of the brightest luminaries of the present century, — what, we ask, is the mortality in the United States, where the veterinary science scarcely has an existence, and where not one man in a hundred can tell a disease of the bowels from one of the lungs? Profiting by the experience of these men, we are in hopes to build up a system of practice that will stand a tower of strength amid the rude shock of medical theories. We have discovered that the lancet is a powerful depressor of vitality, and that poisons derange, instead of producing, healthy action. That they are generally resorted to in this country, no one will deny, and often by men who are unacquainted with the nature of the destructive agents they are making use of.

Hence our business, as reformers, is to expose error, and disseminate true principles. In doing so, we must be guided by the light of reason, and interpret aright the doctrines of nature as they are written by the Creator on the tablets of the whole universe, animate and inanimate.

In our reformed practice, we have true principles to guide us, which no man can controvert; for they are based on the recognition of a curative power in nature, identical with the vital principle, and governed by the same laws that control its action in the healthy state. While, therefore, this system must not change, it may improve; and while it remains on the same foundation, it should progress.

The necessity of aiding nature, in all our modes of medication is the only true principle which should guide us

This we do by the aid of medicines known to be harmless, at the same time paying proper attention to diet, ventilation, exercise, &c., rejecting all processes of cure that depress the vital energy, or destroy the equilibrium of its action.

Our reformed principles teach us that, "Fever is the same in its essential character, under all circumstances and forms which it exhibits. The different kinds, as they are called, are but varieties of the same condition, produced by variations in the prevailing cause, or the strength of vital resistance, or some other peculiarity of the patient. Facts in abundance might be stated to justify this position. Again, fever is not to be regarded as disease, but as a sanative effort; in other words, as an increased or excited state of vital action, whose tendency is to remove from the system any agents or causes that would effect its integrity. Or, perhaps, it might be more properly said, that fever is the effect, or symptom, of accumulated vital action — an index pointing to the progress of causes, operating to ward off disease and restore health.

"Our indications of cure and modes of treatment are to be learned from those manifestations of the vital operations uniformly witnessed in the febrile state. If fever marks the action of the healing power of nature, which we must copy to be successful, why should we not consult the febrile phenomena for our rule of action? Now, what are the indications of cure which we derive from this source? In other words, what are the results which nature designs to accomplish through the instrumentality of fever? They are, an equilibrium of the circulation, a properly-proportioned action of all the organs and an increased depuration of the system, principally by cutaneous evacuations."

Suppose the resistance of some local obstruction, as, for example, an accumulation of partly digested food in the manyplus of the ox, and, for want of a due portion of the gastric fluids to soften the mass and prevent friction, it irritates the mucous covering of the laminæ. The result is inflammation, (local fever,) then general excitement, manifested in an increased state of the circulation generally. The consequences of this general excitement of the mass of the circulation are, a more equal distribution of the blood, and the stimulation of every organ to do a part, according to its capacity, in removing disease. In such cases, the cattle doctors, generally, suppose that the inflammation is confined to the part, (manyplus:) yet it is evident that nature has marshalled her forces and produced a like action on the external surface. How can we prove that this is the case? By the heat, and red surfaces of the membrane lining the nostril, by the accelerated pulse, thirst, &c. Without heat there is no vitality in the system. Now, if the surface be hot, it proves that a large quantity of blood is sent there for the purpose of relieving the deranged internal organ. Hence the reader will perceive, that the cattle doctor whose creed is, "The more fever, the more blood-letting," must be one of the greatest opponents nature has to deal with. Then it is no wonder that so many cattle, sheep and oxen die of fever. The practice of purging, in such a case, would be almost as destructive as the former; for many articles used as purges act on the mucous surfaces of the alimentary canal as mechanical irritants. Nature would, in this case, have to recall her forces from the surface, and concentrate them in the vicinity of parts where they were not wanted, had not man's interference conflicted with her well-planned arrangement, and made her "turn a somerset." When the increased action and heat are manifested on the surface, does it not prove that the different organs are acting harmoniously in self-defence? And is not this action manifested through the same channels in a state of health? Then why call it *disease?*

If obstructions exist as the cause of fever, will the mode of evacuation be different from that of health? Certainly not. Hence the marked tendency of fever to evacuation by the skin or the bowels; the former by perspiration, and the latter by diarrhœa. Fever, then, is a vital action, and the reformers have correct principles. On the other hand, the allopathists tell us that they know very little about fever, but that it is

Our treatment is not directed with a view of combating the fever: we generally aid it by following the indications which it presents; and we often find it necessary, although the surface of the animal shall be hot, and feverish symptoms appear, to use stimulants, (not alcoholic,) combined with antispasmodics and relaxents. (See *Stimulants*, in the APPENDIX.) This class of medicines, aided by warmth and moisture, favors the cutaneous exhalation, and promotes the free and full play of all the functions.

That the allopathist has but few principles to guide him is evident from the following quotations: —

Veterinary surgeon Haycock says, "The profession may flatter itself that it is advancing: for my part, however, I see little or no advancement. Our labors, for the last ten years, have been little more than a repetition of what has gone before. Our books are things of shreds and patches; the system which is followed in the investigation of disease, in the treatment of disease, and in the reporting of it, is altogether so crude and barbarous, that I am thoroughly ashamed of the whole matter.

"I have heard much noise about a *charter*, [which, we presume, means a charter by which men may be licensed to kill *secundum artem*, and '*no questions* ASKED,'] the clamor of which may be compared to the rattling of peas in a dried bladder, or to a storm in a horse-pond. I have also read much which has been said about the *spirit* of this charter. Until I am convinced that it is the best term which can be applied to it, verily the whole is a spirit; for no one, I am persuaded, has ever yet discovered the substance.* It is not charters that

* Mr. White says, "According to the present system of teaching in these chartered institutions, there is very little benefit to be derived by the student."

Mr. Blane experienced in his own person the results of this imperfect system of teaching. He was sent for to fire a valuable horse, and gives the following account of it: "It was my first essay in firing on my own account, and *fired* as I was with my wishes to signalize myself, I labored to enter my novitiate with all due honor. The farrier of the village was ordered to attend, a sturdy old man, civil enough, but looking as though impressed with we want, *but it is that quiet spirit of earnestness which characterizes the true laborer on science.* We require men who will labor for the advancement of the profession from the pure love of the thing; we want, in fact, a few John Fields or men who know how to work and who are possessed of the will to do it."

We hear a great deal said about sending young men from this country to Europe to acquire the principles of the veterinary art, with a view to public teaching. Now, it appears to us that the United States can boast of as great a number of talented physicians, as well qualified to soon learn and understand the fundamental principles of the veterinary art, as their brethren of the old world. There is no country, probably, that can boast of such an amount of talent, in every

no very high respect for a *gentleman farrier's knowledge.* The horse was cast, awkwardly enough, and secured, as will appear, even more so. I, however, proceeded to show the superiority of the new over the old schools. I had just then left the veterinary college, not as a pupil, but as a teacher, which I only mention to mark the climax. On the very first application of the iron, up started my patient, flinging me and my assistants in all directions from him, while he trotted and snorted round the yard with rope, &c. at his heels. As may be supposed, I was taken aback, and might have gone back as I came, had not the old farrier, with much good humor, caught the horse round the neck with his arms, and by some dexterous manœuvre brought him on his knees; when, with a jerk, as quick as unexpected, he threw him at once on his side, when our immediate assistants fixed him, and we proceeded. It is needless to remark that I retired mortified, and left the village farrier lord of the ascendant."

"It cannot be doubted that the best operators in this case are always the common country farriers, who, from devoting themselves entirely to the occupation, soon become proficients."

This admission on the part of a regular graduate of a veterinary institution of London shows that the veterinary science, as taught at the present day, is a matter for reproach. The melancholy triumph of disease over its victims shows that the science is mere moonshine; that, in regard to its most important object, *the cure of disease*, it is mere speculation, rich in theory, but poverty-stricken in its results. Hence we have not only proof that the American people will be immense gainers by availing themselves of the labors of reforms, but, as interested individuals, they have great encouragement to favor our more rational system of treatment. (For additional remarks on this subject, see the author's work on the Horse p. 105.)

department of literature and art, in proportion to the population, as the United States. We know that the veterinary art, with one exception, had its existence from human practitioners, received their fostering care and attention, and grew with their growth. Have we not the materials, then, in this country, to educate and qualify young men to practise this important branch of science? Most certainly. Just send a few to us, for example, and if we do not impart to them a better system of medication than that practised in Europe, by which they will be enabled to treat disease with more success and less deaths, then we will agree to "throw physic to the dogs," and abandon our profession.

The greatest part of the most valuable time of the students of veterinary medicine is devoted to the study of pathology in such a manner as to afford little instruction. For example we are told that in "Bright's" disease of the kidneys they have detected albumen. What does this amount to? Does it throw any rational light on the treatment other than that proposed by us, of toning up the animal, and restoring the healthy secretions? They have studied pathology to their hearts' content; yet any intelligent farmer in this country, with a few simple herbs, can beat them at curing disease. We would give details, were it necessary. Suffice it to say, that it is done here every day, and often through the aid of a little thoroughwort tea, or other harmless agent. The pathologist may discover alterations in tissues, in the blood, and the various organs, and tell us that herein lie the cause and seat of disease; yet these changes themselves are but results, and preceding these were other manifestations of disorder; therefore pathology must always be imperfect, because it is a science of consequences.

The most powerful microscopes have been used to discover the seat of disease; yet this has not taught us to cure one single disease hitherto incurable.

The old school boast that their whole system of blood-letting, purging, and poisoning is based on *enlightened experience* yet their victims have often discovered, by dear-bought "experience," (*many of whom are now doing penance with ulcerated gums, rotten teeth, and fœtid breath,*) that, however valuable this "experience" may be to the M. D.'s, they, the recipients, have not derived that benefit which they were led to expect would accrue to them. From what has already been written in this work, the reader, provided he divests himself of all prejudice, will perceive that allopathic experience is not to be trusted, for their principles are false; hence their experience is also false. Professor Curtis, to whom we are indebted for much valuable information, says, "Do not the old school argue that the most destructive agents in nature may be made to '*aid the vital forces in the removal of disease* by the judicious application of them'? Does not Professor Harrison say, that the lancet is the great anti-inflammatory agent of the *materia medica*, that opium is the *magnum Dei donum* (the great gift of God) for the relief of pain, and that mercury is the great regulator of all the secretions?"

Anatomy and physiology are now being taught in our public schools. The people will, ere long, constitute themselves umpires to decide when doctors disagree. We apprehend it will then be hard work to convince the intelligent and thinking part of the community that poisons and the lancet are sanative agents.

INFLAMMATION.

Inflammation has generally been considered the great bugbear of the old school, and the scarecrow of the cattle doctor. But what do they know about it? Let us see.

Dr. Thatcher says, "Numerous hypotheses or opinions respecting the true nature and cause of inflammation have for ages been advanced, and for a time sustained; but even at the present day, the various doctrines appear to be considered altogether problematical."

Professor Percival says, "Inflammation consists in an increased action of the arteries, and may be either *healthy* or *unhealthy* * — a distinction that appears to relate to some peculiarity of the constitution."

We find inflammation described by most old school authors as disease, and they treat it as such. Professor Payne says, "A great majority of all the disorders to which the human frame is liable begin with inflammation, or end in inflammation, or are accompanied by inflammation in some part of their course, or resemble inflammation in their symptoms. Most of the organic changes in different parts of the body recognize inflammation as their cause, or lead to it as their effect. In short, a very large share of the premature extinctions of human life in general is more or less attributable to inflammation."

The term *inflammation* has long been employed by medical men to denote the existence of an unusual degree of redness, pain, heat, and swelling in any of the textures or organs of which the body is composed. Professor Curtis says, "But as inflammation sometimes exists without the exhibition of any of these symptoms, authors have been obliged to describe it by its causes, in attendant symptoms, and its effects. It is not more strange than true, that, after studying this subject for, *as they say*, four thousand years, experimenting on it and with it, and defining it, the sum of all their knowledge and definitions is this — inflammation in the animal frame is either a simple or compound action, increased or diminished, or a cessation of all action; it either causes, or is caused, or is accompanied, by all the forms of disease to which the body is subject; it is the only agent of cure in every case in which a cure is effected; it destroys all that die, except by accident or old age; it is both disease itself, and the only antidote to disease; it is the pathological principle which lies at the base

* Inflammation is a vital action, and cannot be properly termed *diseased* action. The only action that can be properly termed *diseased* is the chemical action.

of all others; it is that which the profession least of all understand."

Who believes, then, that the science of medicine is based on a sure foundation?

The following selections from the allopathic works will prove what is above stated.

"Pure inflammation is rather an effort of nature than a disease; yet it always implies disease or disturbance, inasmuch as there must be a previous morbid or disturbed state to make such an effort necessary." — *Hunter*, vol. iv. pp. 293, 294.

"As inflammation is an action produced for the restoration of the most simple injury in sound parts which goes beyond the power of union by the first intention, we must look upon it as one of the most simple operations in nature, whatever it may be when arising from disease, or diseased parts. Inflammation is to be considered only a disturbed state of parts, which requires a new but salutary mode of action to restore them to that state wherein a natural mode of action alone is necessary. Therefore inflammation in itself is not to be considered a disease, but a salutary operation consequent either to some violence or to some disease." — *Ibid.* vol. iv. p. 285.

"A wound or bruise cannot recover itself but by inflammation." — *Ibid.* p. 286.

"From whatever cause inflammation arises, it appears to be nearly the same in all; for in all it is an effort intended to bring about a reinstatement of the parts to their natural function." — *Ibid.* p. 286.

Results of Inflammation. — "Inflammation is said to terminate in resolution, effusion, adhesion, suppuration, ulceration, granulation, cicatrization, and mortification. All these different terminations, except the last, may be regarded as so many *vital* processes, exerted in different parts of the animal economy." — *Prof. Thompson*, p. 97.

"Inflammation must needs occupy a large share of attention of both the physician and the surgeon. In nine cases out of ten, the first question which either of them asks himself, on being summoned to the patient, is, *Have I to deal with inflammation here?* It is constantly the object of his treatment and watchful care. It affects all parts that are furnished with bloodvessels, and it affects different parts very variously. . . . . It is by inflammation that wounds are closed and fractures repaired — that parts adhere together when their adhesion is essential to the preservation of the individual, and that foreign and hurtful matters are conveyed out of the body. A cut finger, a deep sabre wound, alike require inflammation to reunite the divided parts. Does ulceration occur in the stomach or intestines, and threaten to penetrate through them — inflammation will often forerun and provide against the danger — glue the threatened membrane to whatever surface may be next it. . . . . The foot mortifies, is killed by injury or by exposure to cold — inflammation will cut off the dead and useless part. An abscess forms in the liver, or a large calculus concretes in the gall-bladder: how is the pus or the calculus to be got rid of? . . . . Partial inflammation precedes and prepares for the expulsion; the liver or the gall-bladder becomes adherent to the walls of the abdomen on the one hand, or to the intestinal canal or the other; and then the surgeon may plunge his lancet into the collection of pus, or the abscess; or the calculus may cut its own way safely out of the body, through the skin or into the bowels." — *Watson*, p. 94.

"The salutary acts of restoration and prevention just adverted to, are such as nature conducts and originates. But we are ourselves able, in many instances, to direct and control the effect of inflammation — nay, we can excite it at our pleasure; and, having excited it, we are able, in a great degree, to regulate its course. And for this reason it becomes, in skilful hands, an instrument of cure." — *Ibid.* p. 94.

The above quotations are not complete. They are selections from the sources whence they are drawn of those portions which testify that fever and inflammation are one and the same thing, and that this same thing consists in a salutary effort of nature to protect the organs of the body from the action of the causes of disease, or to remove those causes and their effects from the organs once diseased. That the same authors teach the very contrary of all this in the same paragraphs, and often in the same sentences, the following extracts will clearly prove: —

Inflammation produces disease. — "When inflammation cannot accomplish that salutary purpose, (a cure,) as in cancer, scrofula, &c., it does mischief." — *Hunter*, p. 285.

"Inflammation is occasionally the cause of disease." — *Ibid.* p. 286.

"In one point of view, it may be considered as a disease itself." — *Ibid.*

"It may be divided into two kinds, the healthy and the unhealthy. . . . The unhealthy admits of a vast variety," &c. — *Ibid.*

"Inflammation often produces mortification or death in the inflamed part." — *Ibid.* vol. iv. p. 305.

"In the light of such authorities, it is surely not strange that no definite knowledge can be obtained of the nature, character, or tendency of inflammation. Of course, no one will dispute the proposition, that medicine, as taught in the schools, is a superstructure without a foundation, and should be wholly rejected." — *Prof. Curtis.*

If the regulars have no correct theory of inflammation, then their system of blood-letting is all wrong. This they acknowledge; for many with whom we have lately conversed say, "We do not use the lancet so often as formerly." One very good reason is, the sovereign people will not let them. Would it not be better for them to abolish its use altogether, as we have done, and avail themselves of the reform of the age?

The following remarks, selected from an address delivered by our respected preceptor, Professor Brown, ought to be read by every friend of humanity.

"The very air groans with the bitter anathemas the people pronounce upon calomel, antimony, copper, zinc, arsenic, arsenious acid, stramonium, foxglove, belladonna, henbane, nux vomica, opium, morphia, and narcotin.

"Hear their bitter cries, borne on every breeze, 'Help! help! help!' See the dim taper of life; it glimmers — 'tis gone! Vitality struggled, and struggled manfully to the last. The poisonous dose was repeated, till the citadel was yielded up.

"The doctor arrives and attempts to comfort and quiet the broken-hearted widow, and helpless, dependent, fatherless children, by recounting the frailties of poor human nature, and reminding them of the fact that all men must die.

"And thus the work of death goes on: the tenderest ties are severed; children are left fatherless; parents are bereaved of their children; families are reduced to fragments; society deprived of her best citizens, and the world filled with misery, confusion, and poverty, in consequence of an evil system of medication. . . .

"The ball is in motion, the banner of medical reform waves gracefully over our beloved country. Hosts of the right stripe are coming to the rescue. Poisons are condemned, the lancet is growing dull, the effusion of blood will soon cease, the battles are half fought, and the victory is sure. . . . While we would have you adhere to the well-established, fundamental principles of reformed medical science, as taught in this school, we would have you recollect that discoveries in knowledge are progressing. . . . . Never entertain the foolish, absurd, and dangerous idea, that because you have been to college, you have learned all that is to be learned — that your education is finished, and you have nothing more to learn. The college is a place where we go to learn how to learn, and the world is the great university, in which our educational exercises terminate with our last expiring breath."

The author craves the reader's indulgence for introducing Dr. Brown's remarks at this stage of the work. It is intended for a class of readers (*the farmers*) who have not the time to make themselves acquainted with all that is going on in the medical world. We aim to make the book acceptable to that class of men. If we fail, the fault is in us, not in our subjects.

REMARKS,

SHOWING THAT VERY LITTLE IS KNOWN OF THE NATURE AND TREATMENT OF DISEASE.

Mr. Percival details a case of peritonitis,* after the usual symptoms in the early stage had subsided. "The horse's bowels became much relaxed: suspecting that there was some disorder in the alimentary canal, and that this was an effort of nature to get rid of it, I promoted the diarrhœa by giving mild doses of cathartic medicine, in combination with calomel!" [Nature did not require such assistance: warm drinks, composed of marshmallows, or slippery elm, would have been just the thing.]

"On the third day from this, prolapsus ani (falling of the fundament) made its appearance. After the return of the gut, the animal grew daily duller, and more dejected, manifesting evident signs of considerable inward disorder, though he showed none of acute pain; the diarrhœa continued; swelling of the belly and tumefaction of the legs speedily followed: eight pounds of blood were drawn, and two ounces of oil of turpentine were given internally, and in spite of another bleeding, and some subordinate measures, carried him off [the treatment, we presume] in the course of a few hours.

"Dissection: a slight blush pervaded the peritoneum; at least the parietal portion of it, for the coats of the stomach and intestines preserved their natural whiteness. About eight gallons of water were measured out of the belly.† The abdominal viscera, as well as the thoracic, showed no marks of disease."

We have stated, in the preceding pages, that the farmers

* Inflammation of the peritoneum.

† Water very frequently accumulates in the belly or chest, after blood-letting.

can generally treat some cases of disease, by simple means, with much better success than some of the regulars; yet there are exceptions. Some of them have been inoculated with the virus of allopathy; and when an animal is taken sick, and manifests evident signs of great derangement, they seem to suppose that the more medicine they cram down the better, forgetting, perhaps not knowing, that the province of the physician is to know when to do nothing. Others err from want of judgment; and if they have an animal sick, they send for the neighbors; each one has a favorite remedy; down go castor oil, aloes, gin and molasses, in rapid succession. "He has inflammation of the insides," says one; "give him salts." No sooner said than done; the salts are hurried down, and, of course, find their way into the paunch. These, together with a host of medicines too numerous to mention are tried without effect: all is commotion within; fermentation commences; gas is evolved; the animal gives signs of woe. As a last resort, paunching, bleeding, &c., follow; perhaps the horns are bored, or some form of barbarity practised, and the animal dies under the treatment.

A case similar to the above came under our notice a few months since. A cow, of a superior breed, was sent a few miles into the country to winter. Having always had the very best of feed, the owner gave particular instructions that she should be fed accordingly; instead of which, however, she was fed on foxgrass and other indigestible matter, in consequence of which she was attacked with acute indigestion, (gastric fever, as it is generally called,) more popularly known, in barn-yard language, as a "stoppage." A man professing to understand *cow-doctoring* was sent for, who, after administering "every thing he could think of" without success, gave a mixture of hog's lard and castor oil. When asked what indication he expected to fulfil, he replied, "My object was to wake up the cow's ideas"! Unfortunately, he awoke the wrong ideas; for the cow died. On making a post mortem examination, about half a bushel of partly-masticated foxgrass was found in the paunch, and the manyplus was distended beyond its physiological capacity. On making an incision into it, the partly-digested food was quite hard and dry, and the mucous covering of the laminæ — even the laminæ themselves — could be detached with the slightest force. The farmer will probably inquire, What ought to be done in such cases? Before we answer the question, a few remarks on the nature of the obstruction seem to be necessary.

In the article *Description of the Organs of Digestion*, the reader will learn the modes by which the food reaches the different compartments of the stomach. In reference to the above case, the causes of derangement are self-evident, which will be seen as we proceed. The animal had, previous to the journey, (thirty miles,) received the greatest care and attention; in short, she had been petted. Being pregnant at the time, the stomach was more susceptible to derangement than at any other time. The long journey could not act otherwise than unfavorably: first, because it would fatigue the muscular system; secondly, because it would irritate the nervous. Here, then, are the first causes; and it is important, in all cases of a deviation from health, to ascertain, as near as possible, the causes, and remove them. *This is considered the first step towards a cure.* If we cannot remove the causes, we are enabled, by an inquiry into them, to adopt the most efficient means for the recovery of the animal. The animal having had a bountiful meal before starting on the journey, and not being allowed sufficient time to remasticate, (rumination is partially or totally suspended during active exercise,) probably, combined with the above causes, an acute attack of the stomach set in — subsided after a few days, and left those organs in a debilitated state. The sudden change in diet also acted unfavorably, especially as the foxgrass required more than ordinary gastric power to reduce it to a pulpy mass, fit to enter the fourth, or true digestive stomach. For want of a due share of vital action in the abomasum, (fourth stomach,) it was unable to perform its part in the physiological process of digestion; hence the accumulation found in the manyplus. The causes of the detachment of laminæ, and the blanched appearances, — for it was as white as new linen, — were partly chemical and partly mechanical. The mechanical obstruction consisted in over-distention of the manyplus from food, thereby obstructing the circulation of the blood through its parietes, (walls,) and depriving it not only of nutriment, from the nerves of nutrition, but paralyzing its secretive function. It then became a prey to chemical action and decomposition. The indications of cure were, to arouse the digestive organs by stimulants, then by anti-spasmodic, relaxing, and tonic medicines, (for which see APPENDIX :) the digestive organs would probably have recommenced their healthy action, and the life of the animal might have been saved. Oil and grease, of every description and kind, are not suitable remedies to administer to cattle when laboring under indigestion; for at best their action is purely mechanical, and cannot be assimilated by the nutritive function so as to act medicinally. Linseed oil is, however, absorbed and diffused. If the animal labors under obstinate constipation, and it is evident that the obstruction is confined to the intestines, then we may resort to a dose of oil.

The reader will perceive the benefits to be derived from a knowledge of animal physiology and veterinary medicine, when based upon sound principles and common sense. He will also see the importance of having educated and honorable men employed in cattle-doctoring. No doubt there are such; but surely something is "rotten in Denmark;" for we are repeatedly told by our patrons that they "judge of the merits of the veterinary art by the men they find engaged in it."

Scientific Treatment of Colic, or Gripes. — "On the 5th September, 1824, a young bay mare was admitted into the infirmary with symptoms of colic, for which she lost eight pounds of blood before she came in. The following drench was prescribed to be given immediately: laudanum and oil of turpentine, of each, three ounces, with the addition of six ounces of decoction of aloes. In the course of half an hour, this was repeated! But shortly after, she vomited the greater part by the mouth and nostrils. No relief having been obtained, twelve pounds of blood were taken from her, and the same drink was given. In another hour, this drench was repeated; and, for the fourth time, during the succeeding hour; both of which, before death, she rejected, as she had done the second drink. Notwithstanding these active measures were promptly taken, she died about three hours after her admission." (See Clark's *Essay on Gripes.*) It appears that the doctors made short work of it. Twelve ounces of laudanum, and the same of turpentine,* in three hours! But this is "*secundum artem*" "skilful treatment" — a specimen of "science and skill," and justifiable in every case where the symptoms are "alarming." Let the reader, if he has ever seen a case of colic treated by us, contrast the result. Had the case been treated with relaxing, anti-spasmodic, carminative drinks, warmth and moisture externally, injections internally, and frictions generally, the poor animal would, probably, have been saved. We have attended many cases of the same sort, and have not yet lost the first one.

Extraordinary case of "cattle doctoring"! — which ought to be termed cattle-killing. — We were requested by Mr. S. of Waltham, December 18, 1850, to see a sick cow. The following is the history of the case: The cow, as near as we could judge, was of native breed, in good condition, and in her eighth pregnant month; pulse, 80 per minute; respirations, 36 per minute; external surface, ears, horns, and legs, cold. She had not dunged for several days. She was found lying on her belly, with her head turned round towards the left side. She struggled occasionally, and appeared to suffer from abdominal pain. She uttered a low, moaning sound when pressure was made on the abdominal muscles. The following facts were related to us by the owner, which we give in his own language: "I bought the cow, and drove her about 200 miles to this place. She had been here about a week, when I perceived she did

* On remonstrating with a man who was about to administer half a pint of turpentine to a cow, he replied, "She has no business to be a cow!" We presume that some of the regulars have just as much, and not a particle more, of the milk of animal kindness as this man seemed to show.

not eat her feed as well as usual. She became sick about nine days ago. I thought it best to begin to doctor her! I employed a man who was reputed to be a pretty good cattle doctor. She got pretty well dosed between us, for we first gave her one pound of salts. The next day we gave her another pound. Finding this also failed to have the desired effect, we gave her one pound eight ounces more. She kept getting worse. We next gave her a quart of urine. She still grew worse. Two table-spoonfuls of gunpowder and a quarter of a pound of antimony were then given; still no improvement. As a last resort, we gave her eight drops of croton oil; a few hours afterwards, nine drops more were given; and a final dose of twenty drops of the same article was administered. The cow rolled her eyes as if she were about to die. I then called in the neighbors to kill her, when one of them advised me to come and see you." The reader will here perceive that we had a pretty desperate case; having been called in just at the eleventh hour. We may here remark that the cow had been under treatment nine days, during which time she had eaten scarcely any food, and passed but very little excrement. The medicine had been given at different stages during that period. There was evidently no accumulation of excrement in the rectum, for she had been raked and received several injections.

As we were not requested to take charge of the case, the owner being unwilling to incur additional expense, we, therefore, with a view of giving present relief, and fulfilling the necessary indications, ordered the following: —

Powdered slippery elm, . . .	1 table-spoonful.
" caraways, ...	1 tea-spoonful.
" marshmallows, . .	1 table-spoonful.
" skullcap, ...	1 tea-spoonful.
" grains of paradise, . .	1 tea-spoonful.

A sufficient quantity of boiling water to form it into the consistence of thin gruel; a junk bottle full to be given every two hours.

Directions were given to rub the ears and extremities until

they were warm, and the strength of the animal to be supported with thin flour gruel.

The indications to be fulfilled were as follows: —

1st. To lubricate the mucous surfaces, and defend them from the action of the drugs.

2d. To arouse the digestive function, and prevent the generation of carbonic acid gas.

3d. To allay nervous excitement, and remove spasms.

Lastly. To equalize the circulation.

The first indication can be fulfilled by slippery elm and marshmallows; the second, by caraway seeds; the third, by skullcap; and the fourth, by grains of paradise.

We have not been able, up to the present time, to ascertain the result.

Here, then, are a few examples of horse and cattle doctoring, which we might multiply indefinitely, did we think it would benefit the reader. We ask the reader to ponder on these facts, and then answer the question, "What do horse and cattle doctors know about the treatment of disease?"

It gives us much pleasure, however, and probably it will the reader, to know that a few of the veterinary surgeons of London are just beginning to see the error of their ways. The following contribution to the Veterinarian, from the pen of Veterinary Surgeon Haycock, will be read with interest. The quotations are not complete. We only select those portions which we deem most instructive to our readers. The disease to which it alludes, *puerperal fever*, has made, and is at the present time making, sad havoc among the stock of our cattle-growing interest; and it stands us in hand to gather honey wherever we can find it. "Of the various questions which present themselves to traders and owners of cattle respecting puerperal fever, the following are, perhaps, a few of the most important: First. At what period of their life are cows the most liable to be attacked with puerperal fever? Secondly At what period after the animal has calved does the disease generally supervene? Thirdly. What is the average rate of mortality amongst cows attacked with this disease? Fourthly

What is the best method to pursue with cattle, in order, if possible, to prevent the disease? Fifthly. What is the best mode of treatment to be pursued with cattle when so attacked? To these several questions I shall endeavor to reply as fully as my own knowledge of the matter will allow me. They are questions which ought to have been answered years ago; [so they would have been, doctor, if, as Curtis says, your brethren had not been *progressing in a circle, instead of direct lines;*] but no one appears to have thought it necessary. They are questions of great importance to the agriculturist; if they were fully answered, he would be able to form a pretty accurate estimate as to the amount of risk he was likely at all times to incur with respect to puerperal diseases of a febrile nature. For instance, suppose it was fully ascertained, from data furnished by the correct observations of a number of practitioners, at what period of the cow's life the animal is most liable to be attacked with puerperal fever; the agriculturist and cow-keeper would be able, in a considerable degree, to guard against it, either by feeding the animal, or taking such other steps as a like experience proved to be the best. It is of no earthly use practitioners writing 'grandiloquent' papers upon diseases like puerperal fever; or in their telling the world, that puerperal fever is a disease of the nervous system; or that the name which is given to it is very improper, *and not suggestive; or that bleeding and the administration of a powerful purgative are proper to commence with;* together with hosts of stereotyped statements of a like nature — statements which are unceasingly repeated, and which are without one jot of sound experience to substantiate them. [All good and sound doctrine.]

"Question First. *At what period of their lives are cows the most liable to be attacked with puerperal fever?* I have in my possession notes and memoranda of twenty-nine cases of this disease, which notes and memoranda I have collected from cases I have treated from the month of July, 1842, to the month of July, 1849 — a period of seven years; and with reference to the above question the figures stand thus: Out of the twenty-nine, three of them were attacked at the third parturient period, five ditto at the fourth, sixteen at the fifth, two at the sixth, and three at the eighth.

"It appears, then, from the above numbers, that cows are the most liable to puerperal fever at the fifth parturient period — a fact which is noticed by Mr. Barlow.

"Secondly. *At what period after the animal has calved does the disease generally supervene?* With reference to this question, the twenty-nine cases stand thus: —

5 cows	immediately after parturition.			
8 "	in 20 hours	"	"	
5 "	in 23	"	"	"
5 "	in 24	"	"	"
3 "	in 30	"	"	"
2 "	in 36	"	"	"
1 "	in 72	"	"	"

"It appears, then, from the above, that after the twentieth and twenty-fourth hours, the animals, comparatively speaking, may be considered as safe from the disease; and that after the seventy-second or seventy-third hour, all danger may be considered as past, beyond doubt.

"Thirdly. *What is the average rate of mortality amongst cows attacked with this disease?* Out of the 29 cases, 12, I find, recovered and 17 died; which loss is equivalent to somewhere about 59 per cent. — a loss which, I am inclined to think, is not so great as that of many other practitioners. [It will be still less if you reject poison as well as the lancet.]

"Mr. Cartwright, in the May number of the Veterinarian of the present year, states that, 'Although I have seen at least a hundred cases, chiefly in this neighborhood, [Whitchurch,] during the last twenty-five years, yet I am almost ashamed to confess that I cannot call to recollection that I ever cured a single case, [neither will you ever cure one as long as the lancet and poison are coöperative,] nor have I ever heard of a case ever being cured by any of the quacks in the neighborhood.' [Of course not, for the quacks follow in the footsteps of their prototypes, the *regular* veterinary surgeons.]

"Fourthly. *What is the best method to pursue with cattle, in order, if possible, to* PREVENT *the disease?* This is a question which I hope to see amply discussed by veterinarians. I have but little to offer respecting it myself; but I labor under a kind of feeling that something valuable may not only be said, but done, by way of prevention. With reference to preventing the disease, Mr. Barlow, in his Essay, says, 'There is a pretty certain preventive in milking the cow some time before calving in full *blood-letting* before or immediately after; in purgatives, very limited diet, and other depletive measures; each and all tending to illustrate the necessity of a vascular state of the system for its development!'"

Mr. Haycock continues: "So far as my own experience is concerned, it is at variance with almost every one of my observations. In the table which I have given respecting question 2, the reader will recollect that I stated that puerperal fever supervened in five cows immediately after parturition. Now, it is worthy of remark, of these five cases, that every animal had been milked many hours previous to calving. The full udder, under such circumstances, is a powerful excitant to the uterus: this is a well-known fact, and the consequence is, that if this natural excitant be withdrawn, the action of the process at once becomes diminished. I have known many cases, in addition to those already given, where the parturient process was prolonged for hours in consequence of the animal's being milked, in whom fever supervened almost immediately afterwards. The prolonged process, I think, greatly weakens the animal, and, as a natural result, the vital energies become less capable of maintaining their normal integrity. With reference, again, to bleeding and purging as preventives, I have nothing to offer in favor of either mode. I do not believe that they are preventives. [Good, again, doctor: you are one of the right stripe. It would give us pleasure to see a few such as you on this side of the water.] First of all, we require to know what percentage of calving cows are liable to be affected with puerperal fever; then, whether that percentage becomes reduced in number in consequence of such preventive measures being brought into force: these are the only modes whereby the matter can be proved; and so far as I know, no one has ever brought the question to such a test. That bleeding and purging are considered as preventives by people in general, I know perfectly; but, like many other popular opinions, the thing which is believed requires first to be proved ere it becomes truth.

"I perfectly agree with Mr. Barlow in recommending spare diet. I regard it, in fact, as the great preventive. . . . . When I say spare diet, I do not mean poor diet. The food should be good, but they should not have that huge bulk of matter which they are capable of devouring, and which they appear so much to desire. I should commence the process for eight or ten days prior to calving, or even, with some animals, much earlier; and the diet I would give should consist of beans, boiled linseed, and boiled oats, with occasionally small portions of hay. I should not always feed upon one mixture. I might occasionally substitute boiled barley in place of oats; and when the time for calving was very near at hand, say within a day or so, I should become more sparing with my hay, and more copious with my allowance of bran. With regard to the diet after calving, I should pursue much the same course I have named: perhaps for the first thirty hours I might allow the animal nothing but gruel and bran mash, in which I should mix a little oatmeal, or very thick gruel. I have sometimes thought — *but hitherto it has not gone beyond a thought with me* — that a broad cotton or linen bandage, fixed moderately tight round the cow's body immediately after calving, might prove of some assistance as a preventive. I have had no experience in its benefit myself; I merely suggest the thing; and if it did nothing more, it would prevent, in some measure, the animal from feeling that sensation of vacuity which must necessarily exist immediately and for some time after calving, and which, I think, under some conditions of the system, may be injurious to the animal. I am told by a medical friend of mine, that he has known puerperal fever produced in women solely from midwives' neglecting to bandage them after delivery; at any rate, a bandage, or a broad belt having straps and buckles attached, and placed securely round the cow's body immediately after calving, and kept there for a day or two, could do no harm, if it failed of doing good.

"Fifthly. *Which is the best method of treatment to pursue with cows when attacked with puerperal fever?* Upon this question I feel that I could say much; but at present I defer its consideration. . . . Suffice it to say, then, that I never either bleed or administer purges. I used once to do both, but my experience has shown me, in numerous cases, that neither is necessary. . . . This malady I have written upon is fearfully destructive; and if such diseases cannot be met with powers capable of wrestling with it, I, for one, shall say that it is a stigma upon our art — I will say that when we are most wanted, we are of the least use."

NATURE, TREATMENT, AND CAUSES OF DISEASE IN CATTLE.

The pathology, or doctrine of diseases, is, as we have previously stated, little understood. Many different causes have been assigned for disease, and as many different modes of cure have been advocated. We shall not discuss either the ancient or modern doctrines any further than we conceive they interfere with correct principles. In doing so, we shall endeavor to confine ourselves to truth, reason, and nature.

We entirely discard the popular doctrine that *fever* and *inflammation* are disease. We look upon them as simple acts of the constitution — sanative in their nature. Then the reader may ask, "Why do you recommend medicine for them?" We do not. We only prescribe medicine, for the purpose of aiding nature to cure the diseases of which *they* (the fever and inflammation) are symptoms, and we do not expect to accomplish even that by medicine alone. Ventilation, diet, and exercise, in nine cases out of ten, will do more good than the destructive agents that have hitherto been used, and christened "cattle medicines."

The great secret of curing diseases is, by accurately observing the indications of nature to carry off and cure disease, and by observing by what critical evacuations she does at last cast off the morbid matter which caused them, and so restores health. By thus observing, following, and assisting *nature*, agreeably to her indications, our practice will always be more satisfactory.

Whenever the great outlets (skin, lungs, and kidneys) of the animal body are obstructed, morbific and excrementitious substances are retained in the system; they irritate, stimulate, and offend nature in such a manner, that she always exerts her power to throw them off. And she acts with great regularity in her endeavors to expel the offending matter, and thus restore the animal to a healthy state.

Suppose an animal to be attacked with disease, and fever supervenes; the whole system is then aroused to cast out this disease: nature invariably points to certain outlets, as the only passages through which the enemy must evacuate the system; and it is the province of the physician to aid in this wise and well-established effort; but when such means are resorted to as in the case of the cow at Waltham, (p. 98,) instead of rendering nature the necessary assistance, her powers and energies are entirely crushed.

Let us suppose a horse to have been exercised; during that exercise, there is a determination of heat and fluids to the surface: the pores of the skin expand and permit the fluids to make their exit: now, if the horse is put into a cold stable, evaporation commences, leaving the surface cold and the pores constricted, so that, after the circulating system has rested a while, it commences a strong action again, to throw off the remaining fluids that were thus suddenly arrested; there is no chance for their escape, as the pores are closed; the skin then becomes dry and harsh, the "coat stares," and the animal has, in common parlance, taken cold, and "it has thrown him into a fever." Now, the cold is the real enemy to be overcome, and the fever should be aided by warmth, moisture, friction, and diffusables. If, at this stage, the cold is removed, the fever will disappear; but if the disease (the cold) has been allowed to advance until a general derangement or sympathetic action is set up, and there is an accumulation of morbific matter in the system, then the restorative process must be more powerful and energetic; constantly bearing in mind that we must assist nature in her endeavors to throw off whatever is the cause of her infirmities. Instead of attacking the disease with the lancet and poison,—which is on the principle of killing the horse to cure the fever,—we should use remedies that are favorable to life. It matters not what organs are affected; the means and processes are the same, and therefore the division of inflammation and fever into a great number of parts designated by as many names, and indicated by twenty times as many complications of symptoms which may never be present, only serve to bewilder the practitioner, and render his practice ineffectual.

PLEURO-PNEUMONIA.

As very little is, at present, known of the nature of this disease, we give the reader the views of Mr. Dun, who received the gold medal offered by the Agricultural Society for the best essay on this subject.

"The causes of the disease, both immediate and remote, are subjects full of interest and importance; and a knowledge of them not only aids in the prevention of disease, but also leads the practitioner to form a more correct prognosis, and to pursue the most approved course of treatment. It is, however, unfortunate that the causes of pleuro-pneumonia have not as yet been satisfactorily explained. No department of the history of the disease is less understood, or more involved in doubt and obscurity. But in this respect pleuro-pneumonia is not peculiar: it is but one of an extensive class which embraces most epidemic and epizoötic diseases. And if the causes which produce influenza, fevers, and cholera, were clearly explained, those which produce pleuro-pneumonia would, in all probability, be easy of solution.

"Viewing the wide-spread and similar effects of pleuro-pneumonia, we may surmise that they are referable to some common cause. And although much difference of opinion exists upon this subject, it cannot be denied that *contagion* is a most active cause in the diffusion of the disease. Indeed, a due consideration of the history and spread of pleuro-pneumonia over all parts of the land will be sufficient to show that, in certain stages of the disease, it possesses the power of infecting animals apparently in a sound and healthy condition, and otherwise unexposed to the action of any exciting cause. The peculiarity of the progress of this disease, from the time that it first appeared in England, is of itself no small evidence of its contagious nature. Its slow and gradual progress is eminently characteristic of diffusion by contagion; and not only were the earlier cases which occurred in this island distinctly proved to have arisen from contact with the Irish droves, but also subsequent cases, even up to the present day, show numerous examples in which contagion is clearly and unequivocally traceable. . . . Although pleuro-pneumonia is not produced by the action of any one of these circumstances alone, [referring to noxious effluvia, &c.,] yet many of them must be considered as predisposing to the disease; and although not its immediate exciting causes, yet, by depressing the physical powers, they render the system more liable to disease, and less able to withstand its assaults. Deficient ventilation, filth, insufficient and bad food, may indeed predispose to the disease, concentrate the animal effluvia, and become the *matrix* and *nidus* of the organic poison; but still, not one, alone, of these circumstances, or even all of them combined, can produce the disease in question. There must be the subtle poison to call them into operation, the specific influence to generate the disease.

"On the other hand, it appears probable that the exciting cause, whether it be contagion, or whatever else, cannot, of itself, generate the disease; but that certain conditions or predisposing causes are necessary to its existence, and without which its specific effects cannot be produced. But although these *remote* or *predisposing* causes are very numerous, they are often difficult of detection; nay, it is sometimes impossible to tell to what the disease is referable, or upon what weak point the exciting cause has fixed itself. A source of perplexity results from the fact. . . . The predisposing causes of the disease admit of many divisions and subdivisions; they may, however, be considered under two general heads — *hereditary* and *acquired*.

"With reference to the former, we know that good points and properties of an animal are transmitted from one generation to another; so also are faults, and the tendencies to particular diseases. As in the same families there is a similarity of external form, so is there also an internal likeness, which accounts for the common nature of their constitution, modified, however, by difference of age, sex, &c.

"Among the acquired predisposing causes of pleuro-pneumonia may be enumerated general debility, local weakness, resulting from previous disease, irritants and stimulants, exposure to cold, damp or sudden changes of temperature, the want of cleanliness, the breathing of an atmosphere vitiated by the decomposition of animal or vegetable matters, or laden with any other impurity. In short, under this head may be included every thing which tends to lower the health and vigor of the system, and consequently to increase the susceptibility to disease.

"The primary symptoms of pleuro-pneumonia are generally obscure, and too often excite but little attention or anxiety. As the disease steals on, the animal becomes dull and dejected, and, if in the field, separates itself from its fellows. It becomes uneasy, ceases to ruminate, and the respirations are a little hurried. If it be a milk-cow, the lacteal secretion is diminished, and the udder is hot and tender. The eyes are dul., the head is lowered, the nose protruded, and the nostrils expanded. The urine generally becomes scanty and high-colored. It is seldom thought that much is the matter with the animal until it ceases to eat; but this criterion does not hold good in most cases of the disease, for the animal at the outset still takes its food, and continues to do so until the blood becomes impoverished and poisoned; it is then that the system becomes deranged, the digestive process impaired, and fever established. The skin adheres to the ribs, and there is tenderness along the spine. Manipulation of the trachea, and percussion applied to the sides, causes the animal to evince pain. Although the beast may have been ill only three days, the number of pulsations are generally about seventy per minute; but they are sometimes eighty and even more. In the first stage, the artery under the jaw feels full and large; but as the disease runs on, the pulse rapidly becomes smaller, quicker, and more oppressed. The breathing is labored, and goes on accelerating as the local inflammation increases. The fore extremities are planted wide apart, with the elbows turned out in order to arch the ribs, and form fixed points for the action of those muscles which the animal brings into operation to assist the respiratory process. In pleuro-pneumonia, the hot stage of fever is never of long duration, [*simply because there is not enough vitality in the system to keep up a continued fever.*] The state of collapse quickly ensues, when the surface heat again decreases, and the pulse becomes small and less distinct. We have now that low typhoid fever so much to be dreaded, and which characterizes the disease in common with epizoötics.

". . . The horse laboring under pleuro-pneumonia, or, indeed, any pulmonary disease, will not lie down; but, in the same circumstances, cattle do so as readily as in health. They do not, however, lie upon their side, but couch upon the sternum, which is broad and flat, and covered by a quantity of fibro-cellular substance, which serves as a cushion; while the articulation between the lower extremities of the ribs admits of lateral expansion of the chest. In this position cattle generally lie towards the side principally affected, thus relieving the sounder side, and enabling it to act more freely. There is sometimes a shivering and general tremor, which may exist throughout the whole course of the disease. (This is owing to a loss of equilibrium between the nerves of nutrition and the circulation.) . . . . As the case advances in severity, and runs on to an unfavorable termination, the pulse loses its strength and becomes quicker. Respiration is in most cases attended by a grunt at the commencement of expiration—a symptom, however, not observable in the horse. The expired air is cold, and of a *noisome* odor. The animal crouches. There is sometimes an apparent knuckling over at the fetlocks, caused by pain in the joints. This symptom is mostly observable in cases when the pleura and pericardium are affected. The animal grinds its teeth. The appetite has now entirely failed, and the emaciation becomes extreme. The muscles, especially those employed in respiration, become wasted; the belly is tucked, and the flanks heave: the oppressive uneasiness is excessive; the strength fails, under the convulsive efforts attendant upon respiration, and the poor animal dies.

"In using means to prevent the occurrence of the disease, we should endeavor to maintain in a sound and healthy tone the physical powers of the stock, and to avoid whatever tends to depress the vital force. Exposure to the influence of contagion [and infection] must be guarded against, and, on the appearance of the disease, every precaution must be used to prevent the healthy having communication with the sick. By a steady pursuance, on the part of the stock proprietor, of these precautionary measures, and by the exercise of care, prudence, and attention, the virulence of the disease will, we are sure be much abated, and its progress checked."

As the reader could not be benefited by our detailing the system of medication pursued in England,—at least we should judge not, when we take into consideration the great loss that attends their *best efforts*,—we shall therefore proceed to inform the reader what the treatment ought to be in the different stages of the disease.

General Indication of Cure in Pleuro-Pneumonia. — Restore the suppressed evacuations, or the secretions and excretions, if they are obstructed.

If bronchial irritation or a cough be present, shield and defend the mucous surfaces from irritation. Relieve congestions by equalizing the circulation. Support the powers of the system. Relieve all urgent symptoms.

Special Practice. — Suppose a cow to be attacked with a slight cough. She appears dull, and is off her feed; pulse full, and bowels constipated; and she is evidently out of condition.

Then the medicines should be anti-spasmodic and relaxent, tonic, diaphoretic, and lubricating.

The following is a good example: —

Powdered golden seal, (tonic,) . . .	1 table-spoonful.
" mandrake, (relaxent,) . .	2 tea-spoonfuls.
" lobelia, (anti-spasmodic,) .	1 tea-spoonful.
" slippery elm or mallows, (lubricating,) . . .	1 table-spoonful.
" hyssop tea, (diaphoretic,) .	1 gallon.

After straining the hyssop tea, mix with it the other ingredients, and give a quart every two hours.

In the mean time, administer the following injection: —

Powdered lobelia, ...	of each, half a
" ginger, ...	table-spoonful.
Boiling water, ...	1 gallon.

When cool, inject.

Particular attention must be paid to the general surface. If the surface and the extremities are cold, then employ friction, warmth, and moisture. The animal must be in a comfortable barn, neither too hot nor too cold; if it be imperfectly ventilated, the atmosphere may be improved by stirring a red-hot iron in vinegar or pyroligneous acid, or by pouring either of these articles on heated bricks. The strength is to be supported, provided the animal be in poor condition, with gruel, made of flour and shorts, equal parts; but, as it frequently happens (in this country) that animals in good flesh are attacked, in such case food would be inadmissible.

Suppose the animal to have been at pasture, and she is not observed to be "ailing" until rumination is suspended. She then droops her head, and has a cough, accompanied with difficult breathing, weakness in the legs, and sore throat. Then, in addition to warmth, moisture, and friction, as already directed, apply to the joints and throat the following: —

Boiling vinegar, ...	1 quart.
African cayenne, ...	1 table-spoonful.

The throat being sore, the part should be rubbed gently. The joints may be rubbed with energy for several minutes. The liquid must not be applied too hot.

Take

Virginia snakeroot, . . .	of each, 2 ounces.
Sage, ...	
Skullcap, (herb,)	1 ounce.
Pleurisy root, ...	1 ounce.
Infuse in boiling water, ...	1 gallon.

After standing for the space of one hour, strain; then add a gill of honey and an ounce of powdered licorice or slippery elm. Give a quart every four hours.

Should the cough be troublesome, give

Balsam copaiba, ...	1 table-spoonful.
Sirup of garlic, ...	1 ounce.
Thin gruel, ...	1 quart.

Give the whole at a dose, and repeat as occasion may

require. A second dose, however, should not be given until twelve hours have elapsed.

Injections must not be overlooked, for several important indications can be fulfilled by them. (For the different forms, see APPENDIX.)

If the disease has assumed a typhus form, then the indications will be, —

First. To equalize the circulation and nervous system, and maintain that equilibrium. This is done by giving the following: —

Powdered African cayenne, . .	1 tea-spoonful.
" flagroot, ...	1 table-spoonful.
Skullcap, ...	$\frac{1}{2}$ ounce.
Marshmallows, ...	4 ounces.

Put the whole of the ingredients into a gallon of water; boil for five minutes; and, when cool, strain; sweeten with a small quantity of honey; then give a quart every two hours.

The next indication is, to counteract the tendency to putrescence. This may be done by causing the animal to inhale the fumes of pyroligneous acid, and by the internal use of bayberry bark. They are both termed antiseptics. The usual method of generating vapor for inhalation is, by first covering the animal's head with a horse-cloth, the corners of which are suffered to fall below the animal's nose, and held by assistants in such a manner as to prevent, as much as possible, the escape of the vapor. A hot brick is then to be grasped in a pair of tongs, and held about a foot beneath the nose. An assistant then pours the acid, (*very gradually,*) on the brick. Half a pint of acid will be sufficient for one steaming, provided it be used with discretion; for if too much is poured on the brick at once, the temperature will be too rapidly lowered.

In reference to the internal use of bayberry, it may be well to remark, that it is a powerful astringent and antiseptic, and should always be combined with relaxing, lubricating medicines. Such are licorice and slippery elm.

The following may be given as a safe and efficient antiseptic drink: —

Powdered bayberry bark, .	half a table-spoonful.
" charcoal, . . .	1 table-spoonful
Slippery elm, ...	1 ounce
Boiling water, ...	1 gallon.

Mix. Give a quart every two hours.

The diet should consist of flour gruel and boiled carrots. Boiled carrots may be allowed (provided the animal will eat them) during the whole stage of the malady.

The object of these examples of special practice is to direct the mind of the farmer at once to something that will answer a given purpose, without presuming to say that it is the best in the world for that purpose. The reader will find in our *materia medica* a number of articles that will fulfil the same indications just as well.

LOCKED-JAW.

Mr. Youatt says, "Working cattle are most subject to locked-jaw, because they may be pricked in shoeing; and because, after a hard day's work, and covered with perspiration, they are sometimes turned out to graze during a wet or cold night. Over-driving is not an uncommon cause of locked-jaw in cattle. The drovers, from long experience, calculate the average mortality among a drove of cattle in their journey from the north to the southern markets; and at the head of the list of diseases, and with the greatest number of victims, stands 'locked-jaw,' especially if the principal drover is long absent from his charge."

The treatment of locked-jaw, both in horses and cattle, has, hitherto, been notoriously unsuccessful. This is not to be wondered at when we take into consideration the destructive character of the treatment.

"Take," says Mr. Youatt, "twenty-four pounds of blood from the animal; or bleed him almost to fainting. . . . Give him Epsom salts in pound and a half doses (!) until it operates. Purging being established, an attempt must be made to allay the irritation of the nervous system by means of sedatives; and the best drug is opium.* The dose should be a drachm three times a day. [One fortieth part of the quantity here recommended to be given in one day would kill a strong man who was not addicted to its use.] At the same time, the action of the bowels must be kept up by Epsom salts, or common salt, or sulphur, and the proportion of the purgative and the sedative must be so managed, that the constitution shall be under the influence of both.† A seton of black hellebore root may be of service. It frequently produces a great deal of swelling and inflammation.‡ . . . If the disease terminates successfully, the beast will be left sadly out of condition, and he will not thrive very rapidly. He must, however, be got into fair plight, as prudence will allow, and then sold; for he will rarely stand much work afterwards, or carry any great quantity of flesh." The same happens to us poor mortals when we have been dosed *secundum artem.* We resemble walking skeletons.

Our own opinion of the disease is, that it is one of nervous origin, and that the tonic spasm, always present in the muscles

* This is a narcotic vegetable poison; and although large quantities have been occasionally given to the horse without apparent injury, experience teaches us that poisons in general — notwithstanding the various modes of their action, and the difference in their symptoms — all agree in the abstraction of vitality from the system. Dr. Eberle says, "Opiates never fail to operate perniciously on the whole organization." Dr. Gallup says, "The practice of using opiates to mitigate pain is greatly to be deprecated. It is probable that opium and its preparations have done seven times the injury that they have rendered benefit on the great scale of the civilized world Opium is the most destructive of all narcotics."

† This is a perfect seesaw between efforts to kill and efforts to cure.

‡ Then it ought not to be used.

of voluntary motion, is only symptomatic of derangement in the great, living electro-galvanic battery, (the brain and spinal cord,) or in some of its wires (nerves) of communication.

Mr. Percival says, "Tetanus consists, in a spasmodic contraction, more or less general, of the muscles of voluntary motion, and especially of those that move the lower jaw; hence the vulgar name of it, *locked-jaw*, and the technical one of *trismus*."

In order to make ourselves clearly understood, and furnish the reader with proper materials for him to prosecute his inquiries with success, a few remarks on the origin of muscular motion seem to be absolutely necessary.

It is generally understood by medical men, and taught in the schools, that there are in the animal economy four distinct systems of nerves.

1st system. This consists of the sensitive nerves, which are distributed to all parts of the animal economy endowed with feeling; and all external impulses are reflected to the medulla oblongata, &c. (See *Dadd's work on the Horse*, p. 127.) In short, these nerves are the media through which the animal gets all his knowledge of external relations.

2d system. The motive. These proceed from nearly the same centre of perception, and distribute themselves to all the muscles of voluntary motion. It is evident that the muscle itself cannot perform its office without the aid of the nerves, (electric wires;) for it has been proved by experiment on the living animal, that when the posterior columns of nervous matter, which pass down from the brain towards the tail, are severed, then all voluntary motion ceases. Motion may, however, continue; but it can only be compared to a ship at sea without a rudder, having nothing to direct its course. It follows, then, that if the nerves of motion and sensation are severed, there is no communication between the parts to which they are distributed and the brain. And the part, if its nutritive function be also paralyzed, will finally become as insensible as a stone — wither and die.

3d system. The respiratory. These are under the control of

the will only through the superior power, as manifested by the motive nerves. For the animal will breathe whether it wishes to or not, as long as the vital spark burns.

4th system. The sympathetic, sometimes called *nutritive nerves.* They are distributed to all the organs of digestion, absorption, circulation, and secretion. These four nervous structures, or systems, must all be in a physiological state, in order to carry on, with unerring certainty, their different functions. If they are injured or diseased, then the perceptions of external relations are but imperfectly conveyed to the mind. (*Brutes have a mind.*) On the other hand, if the brain, or its appendages, spinal marrow, &c., be in a pathological state, then the manifestations of *mind* or *will* are but imperfectly represented. Now, it is evident to every reasonable man, that the nerves may become diseased from various causes; and this explains the reason why locked-jaw sometimes sets in without any apparent cause. The medical world have then agreed to call it *idiopathic.* This term only serves to bewilder us, and fails to throw the least light on the nature of the malady, or its causes. Many men ridicule the idea of the nerves being diseased, just because alterations in their structure are not evident to the senses. We cannot see the atoms of water, nor even the myriads of living beings abounding in a single drop of water! yet no one doubts that water contains many substances imperceptible to the naked eye. We know that epizoötic diseases are wafted, by the winds, from one part of the world to another; yet none of us have ever seen the specific virus. Can any man doubt its existence?

Hence it appears that diseases may exist in delicately-organized filaments, without the cognizance of our external perceptions.

It is further manifest that locked-jaw is only symptomatic of diseased nervous structures, and that a pathological state of the nervous filaments may be brought about independent of a prick of a nail, or direct injury to a nerve.

Hence, instead of tetanus consisting "in a spasmodic contraction of the muscles of voluntary motion," it consists in a deranged state of the nervous system, and the contracted state of the muscles is only symptomatic of such derangement. Then what sense is there in blistering, bleeding, and inserting setons in the dewlap? Of what use is it to treat symptoms? Suppose a man to be attacked with hepatitis, (inflammation of the liver:) he has a pain in the right shoulder. Suppose the physician prescribes a plaster for the latter, without ascertaining the real cause, or perhaps not knowing of its existence. We should then say that the doctor only treated symptoms. "And he who treats symptoms never cures disease." Suppose locked-jaw to have supervened from an attack of acute indigestion: would it not be more rational to restore the lost function?

Suppose locked-jaw to have set in from irritating causes, such as bots in the stomach, worms in the intestines, &c.: would bleeding remove them? would it not render the system less capable of recovering its physiological equilibrium, and resisting the irritation produced by these animals on the delicate nervous tissues?

Suppose, as Mr. Youatt says, that locked-jaw sets in "after turning the animal out to graze during a cold night:" will a blister to the spine, or a seton in the dewlap, restore the lost function of the skin?

In short, would it not be more rational, in cases of locked-jaw, to endeavor to restore the healthy action of all the functions, instead of depressing them with the agents referred to?

Then the question arises, What are the indications to be fulfilled?

First. Restore the lost function.

Secondly. Equalize the circulation, and maintain an equilibrium between nervous and arterial action.

Thirdly. Support the powers of life.

Fourthly. If locked-jaw arise from a wound, then apply suitable remedial agents to the part, and rescue the nervous system from a pathological state.

To fulfil the fourth indication, we commence the treatment as follows:—

Suppose the foot to have been pricked or wounded. We

make an examination of the part, and remove all extraneous matter. The following poultice must then be applied:—

Powdered skunk cabbage, " lobelia, . . " poplar bark, .	. . equal parts.
Indian meal, ...	1 pint.

Make it of the proper consistence with boiling water. When sufficiently cool, put it into a flannel bag, and secure it above the pastern. To be renewed every twelve hours. After the second application, examine the foot, and if suppuration has commenced, and matter can be felt, or seen, a small puncture may be made, taking care not to let the knife penetrate beyond the bony part of the hoof.

In the mean time, prepare the following drink:—

Indian hemp or milkweed, (herb,) .	1 ounce.
Powdered mandrake, ...	1 table-spoonful.
Powdered lobelia seeds, ...	1 tea-spoonful.
" poplar bark, (very fine,) .	1 ounce.

Make a tea, in the usual manner — about one gallon. After straining it through a cloth, add the other ingredients, and give a quart every two hours.

A long-necked bottle is the most suitable vehicle in which to administer; but it must be poured down in the most gradual manner. The head should not be elevated too high.

A liberal allowance of camomile tea may be resorted to, during the whole stage of the disease.

Next stimulate the external surface, by warmth and moisture, in the following manner: Take about two quarts of vinegar, into which stir a handful of lobelia; have a hot brick ready, (*the animal having a large cloth, or blanket, thrown around him;*) pour the mixture gradually on the brick, which is held over a bucket to prevent waste; the steam arising will relax the surface. After repeating the operation, apply the following mixture around the jaws, back, and extremities: take of cayenne, skunk cabbage, and cypripedium, (lady's slipper,) powdered, each two ounces, boiling vinegar two quarts; stir the mixture until sufficiently cool, rub it well in with a coarse sponge; this will relax the jaws a trifle, so that the animal can manage to suck up thin gruel, which may be given warm, in any quantity. This process must be persevered in; although it may not succeed in every case, yet it will be more satisfactory than the blood-letting and poisoning system. No medicine is necessary; the gruel will soften the fæces sufficiently; if the rectum is loaded with fæces, give injections of an infusion of lobelia.

INFLAMMATORY DISEASES.

INFLAMMATION OF THE STOMACH, (Gastritis.)

Such a complicated piece of mechanism is the stomach of the ox, that that organ is particularly liable to disease. Inflammation, being the same as local fever, (or a high grade of vital power, concentrated within a small space,) may be produced by over-feeding, irritating and indigestible food, or acrid, poisonous, and offensive medicines. The farmer must remember that a small quantity of good, nutritious food, capable of being easily penetrated by the gastric fluids, will repair the waste that is going on, and improve the condition with more certainty than an abundance of indifferent provender.

Cure. — The first indication will be to allay the irritability of the stomach; this will moderate the irritation and lessen the fever. Make a mucilaginous drink of slippery elm, or marshmallows, and give half a pint every two hours. All irritating food and drink must be carefully avoided, and the animal must be kept quiet; all irritating cordials, "including the popular remedy, gin and molasses," must be avoided. These never fail to increase the malady, and may occasion death. If there is an improper accumulation of food in the viscera, the remedies will be, relaxing clysters, abstinence from food, and a tea of sassafras and mandrake, made thus: —

Sassafras, (*laurus sassafras*,)	1 ounce.
Mandrake, (*podophyllum peltatum*,) . .	4 drachms.
Boiling water.	2 quarts.

Let the mixture stand until quite cool, and give a pint every four hours.

Almost all animals, when suffering under acute symptoms, require diluting, cooling drinks. This at once points out the use of water, or any weak gruel of which water is the basis; the necessity of diluting liquors is pointed out by the heat and dryness of the mouth, and rigidity of the coat.

When the thirst is great, the following forms a grateful and cooling beverage: Take lemon balm, (*melissa officinalis*,) two ounces; boiling water, two quarts; when cool, strain, and add half a tea-spoonful of cream of tartar. Give half a pint at intervals of two hours.

If the stomach continues to exhibit a morbid state, which may be known by a profuse discharge of saliva from the mouth, then administer camomile tea in small quantities; the addition of a little powdered charcoal will prove beneficial.

Remarks. — Gastritis cannot be long present without other parts of the system sharing the disturbance: it is then termed gastric fever. This fever is the result of the local affection. Our object is, to get rid of the local affection, and the fever will subside. Authors have invariably recommended destructive remedies for the cure of gastritis; but they generally fail of hitting the mark, and always do more or less injury.

A light diet, rest, a clean bed of straw in a well-ventilated barn, will generally perfect the cure.

INFLAMMATION OF THE LUNGS, (PNEUMONIA.)

Causes. — Errors in feeding, over-exertion, exposure in wet pastures, or suffering the animal, when in a state of perspiration, to partake too bountifully of cold water, are among the direct causes of a derangement of vital equilibrium. Want of pure air for the purpose of vitalizing the blood, the inhalation of noxious gases, and filth and uncleanliness, may produce this disease in its worst form; yet it must be borne in mind that the same exciting causes will not develop the same form of disease in all animals. It altogether depends on the amount of vital resistance, or what is termed the peculiar idiosyncrasy of the animal. On the other hand, several animals often suffer from the same form of disease, from causes varying in their general character. Hence the reader will see that it would be needless, in fact impossible, to point to the direct cause in each grade of disease. The least obstruction to universal vital action will produce pneumonia in some animals, while in others it may result in disease of the bowels.

Cure. — No special treatment can be successfully pursued in pneumonia; for the lungs are not the only organs involved: no change of condition can occur in the animal functions without the nervous system being more or less deranged; for the latter is essential to all vital motions. Hence disease, in every form, should be treated according to its indications. A few general directions may, however, be found useful. The first indication to be fulfilled is to equalize the blood. Flannels saturated with warm vinegar should be applied to the extremities; they may be folded round the legs, and renewed as often as they grow cold. Poultices of slippery elm, applied to the feet, as hot as the animal can bear them, have sometimes produced a better result than vinegar. If the animal has shivering fits, and the whole surface is chilled, apply warmth and moisture as recommended in article "*Locked-Jaw.*" At the same time, endeavor to promote the insensible perspiration by the internal use of diaphoretics — ***lobelia or thoroughwort tea.*** A very good diaphoretic and anti-spasmodic drink may be made thus: —

Lobelia, (herb,)	2 ounces.
Spearmint, ...	1 ounce.
Boiling water, ...	2 quarts.

Let the above stand for a few minutes; strain, then add two table-spoonfuls of honey. Give half a pint every hour, taking care to pour it down the œsophagus very gently, so as to insure its reaching the fourth or true digestive stomach. The following clyster must be given:—

Powdered lobelia, ...	2 ounces.
Boiling water, ...	3 quarts.

When sufficiently cool, inject with a common metal syringe.

These processes should be repeated as the symptoms require, until the animal gives evidence of relief; when a light diet of thin gruel will perfect the cure. It must ever be borne in mind that in the treatment of all forms of disease—those of the *lungs more especially*—the animal must have pure, uncontaminated atmospheric air, and that any departure from purity in the air which the animal respires, will counteract all our efforts to cure.

INFLAMMATION OF THE BOWELS, (ENTERITIS.—INFLAMMATION OF THE FIBRO-MUSCULAR COAT OF THE INTESTINES.)

Character.—Acute pain; the animal appears restless, and frequently turns his head towards the belly; moans, and appears dull; frequent small, hard pulse; cold feet and ears.

Causes.—Plethora, costiveness, or the sudden application of cold either internally or externally, overworking, &c.

Cure.—In the early stages of the disease, all forms of medication that are in any way calculated to arouse the peristaltic motion of the intestines should be avoided; hence purges are certain destruction. Relax the muscular structure by the application of a blanket or horse-cloth wrung out in hot water. In this disease, it is generally sufficient to apply warmth and moisture as near the parts affected as possible; yet if the ears and legs are cold, the general application of warmth and moisture will more speedily accomplish the relaxation of the whole animal. After the application of the above, injections of a mild, soothing character (slippery elm, or flaxseed tea) should be used very liberally. A drink of any mucilaginous, lubricating, and innocent substance may be given, such as mallows linseed, Iceland moss, slippery elm. During convalescence, the diet must be light and of an unirritating character, such as boiled carrots, scalded meal, &c.

INFLAMMATION OF THE PERITONEAL COAT OF THE INTESTINES, (Peritonitis.)

This disease requires the same treatment as the latter malady.

INFLAMMATION OF THE KIDNEYS, (Nephritis.)

The usual symptoms are a quick pulse ; loss of appetite high-colored urine, passed in small quantities, with difficulty and pain. Pressure on the loins gives pain, and the animal will shrink on placing the hand over the region of the kidneys.

Causes. — Cold, external injury, or injury from irritating substances, that are often sent full tilt through the kidneys, as spirits of turpentine, gin and molasses, saleratus. It is unnecessary to detail all the causes of the disease : suffice it to say, that they exist in any thing that can for a time obstruct the free and full play of the different functions.

Treatment. — This, too, will consist in the invitation of the blood to the surface and extremities, and by removing all irritating matter from the system, *in the same manner as for inflammation of the bowels.* The application of a poultice of ground hemlock, or a charge of gum hemlock, will generally be found useful. The best drinks — and these should only be allowed in small quantities — are gum arabic and marshmallow decoctions.

INFLAMMATION OF THE BLADDER, (Cystitis.)

During the latter months of pregnancy, the bladder is often in an irritable state, and a frequent desire to void the urine is observed, which frequently results from constipation. A peculiar sympathy exists between the bladder and rectum; and when constipation is present, there is a constant effort on the part of the animal to void the excrement. This expulsive action also affects the bladder: hence the frequent efforts to urinate. The irritable state of the bladder is caused by the pressure of the loaded rectum on the neck of the former.

The common soap-suds make a good injection, and will quickly soften the hardened excrement; after which the following clyster may be used:—

Linseed tea, ...	3 quarts.
Cream of tartar, ...	1 ounce.

After throwing into the rectum about one third of the above, press the tail on the anus. The object is, to make it act as a fomentation in the immediate vicinity of the parts. After the inflammation shall have subsided, administer the following in a bottle, or horn:—

Powdered blackroot, (*leptandra virginica,*)	half an ounce.
Warm water, ...	1 pint.

Repeat the dose, if the symptoms are not relieved.

INFLAMMATION OF THE WOMB.

This may be treated in the same manner as the last-named disease. The malady may be recognized by lassitude, loss of appetite, diminution in the quantity, and deterioration in the quality, of the milk. As the disease advances, there is often a fetid discharge from the parts; a constant straining, which is attended with a frequent flow of urine.

INFLAMMATION OF THE BRAIN, (PHRENITIS.)

In this disease, the pia mater, arachnoid membrane, or the brain itself, may be inflamed. It matters very little which of the above are deranged, for the means of cure are the same. We have no method of making direct application to either of the above, as they all lie within the cranium. Neither can we act upon them medicinally except through the organs of secretion, absorption, and circulation. Post mortem examinations reveal to us evident marks of high inflammatory action, both in the substance of the brain and in its membranes; and an effusion of blood, serum, or of purulent matter, has been found in the ventricles of the brain.

Treatment. — The indications are, to equalize the circulation by warmth and moisture externally, and maintain the action to the surface by rubbing the legs with the following counter-irritant: —

Vinegar, ...	1 quart.
Common salt, ...	2 ounces.

Set the mixture on the fire, (*in an earthen vessel,*) and allow it to simmer for a few moments; then apply it to the legs. After the circulation is somewhat equalized, give the following drench: —

Extract of butternut, . . .	half an ounce.
Tea of hyssop, ...	1 pint.

A stimulating clyster may then be given, composed of warm water, into which a few grains of powdered capsicum may be sprinkled.

If due attention be paid to counter-irritation, and the head kept cool by wet cloths, the chances of recovery are pretty certain.

INFLAMMATION OF THE EYE.

This disease is too well known to require any description; we shall therefore, at once, proceed to point out the ways and means for its cure.

Treatment. — First wash the eyes with a weak decoction of camomile flowers until they are well cleansed; then give a cooling drink, composed of

Cream of tartar, ...	1 ounce.
Decoction of lemon balm, . . .	1 quart.

Repeat this drink every six hours, until the bowels are moved. Should the disease occur where these articles cannot be procured, give two ounces of common salt in a pint of water. Should the eye still continue red and swollen, give a dose of physic. (See *Physic for Cattle.*)

If a film can be observed, wash with a decoction of powdered bloodroot; and if a weeping remain, use the following astringent: —

Powdered bayberry bark, ...	1 ounce.
Boiling water, ...	1 pint.

When cool, pour off the clear liquor. It is then fit for use. Inflammation of the eye may assume different forms, but the above treatment, combined with attention to rest, ventilation, a dark location, and a light diet, will cover the whole ground.

INFLAMMATION OF THE LIVER, (HEPATITIS.)

Cattle very frequently show signs of diseased liver. Stall-fed oxen and cows kept in cities are most liable to derangement of the liver; in such animals, (after death,) there is an unusual yellowness of the fat. A disease of the liver may exist for a long time without interfering much with the genera. health. Mr. Youatt informs us that "a chronic form of diseased liver may exist for some months, or years, not characterized by any decided symptom and but little interfering with health."

Symptoms. — Permanent yellowness of the eyes; quick pulse; dry muzzle; hot mouth; considerable pain when pressure is made on the right side. Occasionally the animal looks round and licks the spot over the region of the liver.

Treatment. — First give half pint doses of thoroughwort tea, at intervals of one hour, (*to the amount of two quarts.*) This will relax the system, and equalize vital action. The following drench is then to be given: —

Extract of butternut, ...	half an ounce.
Warm water, ...	1 quart.

If the butternut cannot be obtained, substitute a dose of physic. (See APPENDIX.) Stimulate the bowels to action by injections of soap-suds. If the extremities are cold, proceed to warm them in the manner alluded to in article *Inflammation of the Bowels.* On the other hand, if the surface of the body is hot and dry, and there is much fever present, indicated by a quick pulse and dry muzzle, then bathe the whole surface with weak saleratus water, sufficiently warm to relax the external surface. The following fever drink may be given daily until rumination again commences: —

Lemon balm, ...	2 ounces.
Cream of tartar, ...	1 ounce.
Honey, ...	1 gill.
Water, ...	2 quarts.

First pour the boiling water on the balm; after standing a few minutes, strain; then add the above ingredients.

JAUNDICE, OR YELLOWS.

This disease is well known to every farmer; the yellow appearance of the skin, mouth, eyes, and saliva at once betray its presence. It consists in the absorption of unchanged bile into the circulation, which bile becomes diffused, giving rise to the yellow appearances.

In the treatment of jaundice, we first give a dose of physic, (see Appendix,) and assist its operation by injections of weak lie, made from wood ashes. The animal may roam about in the barn-yard, if the weather will permit; or rub the external surface briskly with a wisp or brush, which will answer the same purpose. The following may be given in one dose, and repeated every day, or every other day, as the symptoms may require:—

Powdered golden seal, (*hydrastus canadensis*,) . .	1 table-spoonful.
" slippery elm, ...	2 ounces.

Water sufficient to make it of the consistence of gruel.

Should a diarrhœa set in, it ought not to occasion alarm, but may be considered as an effort of nature to rid the system of morbific matter. It will be prudent, however, to watch the animal, and if the strength and condition fail, then add to the last prescription a small quantity of powdered gentian and caraway seeds.

There are various forms of disease in the liver, yet the treatment will not differ much from that of the last-named disease. There is no such thing as a medicine for a particular symptom, in one form of disease, that is not equally good for the same symptom in every form. In short, there is no such thing as a specific. Any medicine that will promote the healthy action of the liver in one form of jaundice will be equally good for the same purpose in another form of that disease.

Mr. Youatt states, "There are few diseases to which cattle

are so frequently subject, or which are so difficult to treat, as jaundice, or yellows." Hence it is important that the farmer should know how and in what manner the disease may be prevented. And he will succeed best who understands the causes, which often exist in overworking the stomach, with a desire to fatten. Men who raise cattle for the market often attempt to get them in fine condition and flesh, without any regard to the state of the digestive organs, the liver included; for the bile which the latter secretes is absolutely necessary for the perfection of the digestive process. They do not take into consideration the state of the animals' health, the climate, the quality of food, and the quantity best adapted to the digestive powers; and what is of still greater importance, and too often overlooked, is, that all animals should be fed at regular intervals. Some men suppose that so long as their cattle shall have good food, without any regard to quantity, — if they eat all day long, and cram their paunch to its utmost capacity, — they must fatten; when, in fact, too much food deranges the whole digestive apparatus. As soon as the paunch and stomach are overloaded, they press on the liver, interfering with the bile-secreting process, producing congestion and disorganization.

Diseases of the liver may be produced by any thing that will for a time suspend the process of rumination: the known sympathy that exists between the stomach and liver explains this fact.

Digestion, like every other vital process, requires a concentration of power to accomplish it: now, if an ox should have a bountiful meal, and then be driven several miles, the process of digestion, during the journey, will be partly suspended. The act of compelling an ox to rise, or annoying him in any way, will immediately suspend rumination, which may result in an acute disease of the liver. In most cases, however, the stomach is primarily affected.

Dealers in cattle often overfeed the animals they are about to dispose of, in order to improve their external appearance, and increase their own profits: the consequence is, that such animals are in a state of plethora, and are liable at any moment to be attacked with congestion of the liver or brain.

Again. If oxen are driven a long journey, and then turned into a pasture abounding in highly nutritious grasses or clover, to which they are unaccustomed, they fill the paunch to such an extent that it becomes a matter of impossibility on the part of the animal to throw it up for rumination; this mass of food, being submitted to the combined action of heat and moisture, undergoes fermentation; carbonic acid gas is evolved; the animal is then said to be "blown," "hoven," or "blasted." Post mortem examination, in such cases, reveals a highly-congested state of the liver and spleen.

In fattening cattle, the injury done to the organs of digestion is not always observed in the early stages; for the vital power, which wages a warfare against all encroachments, endeavors to accommodate itself to the increased bulk; yet, by continuing to give an excess of diet, it finally yields up the citadel to the insidious foe. Chemical action then overpowers the vital, and disease is the result.

Thousands of valuable cattle are yearly destroyed by being too well, or, rather, injudiciously fed. Many diseases of the liver and digestive organs result from feeding on unwholesome, innutritious, and hard, indigestible food. Bad water, and suffering the animal to partake too bountifully of cold water when heated and fatigued, are among the direct causes of disease.

DISEASES OF THE MUCOUS SURFACE.

The mucous membrane is a duplicature of the skin, and is folded into the external orifices of the animal, as the mouth, ears, nose, lungs, stomach, intestines, and bladder; but not being so much exposed to the action of external agents, it is not so strong or thick as the skin. It performs, however, nearly the same office as the skin. If the action of one is suppressed, the other immediately commences the performance of its office. Thus a common cold, which collapses the skin, immediately stops insensible perspiration, which recedes to the mucous membrane, producing a discharge from the nose, eyes, bowels, &c. So, when great derangement of the mucous membrane exists, debilitating perspiration succeeds. In the treatment of diseases of the mucous membrane, we endeavor to remove the irritating causes from the organs affected, restore the general tone of the system, and invite action to the external surface.

CATARRH, OR HOOSE.

This disease often arises from exposure to wet or cold weather, and from the food being of a bad quality, or deficient in quantity. If the animal is enfeebled by poor feed, old age, or any other cause, then there is very little resistance offered against the encroachments of disease: hence young beasts and cows after calving are often the victims.

Treatment.—It is necessary to attend to this disorder as soon as it makes its appearance; for a common cold, neglected, often lays the foundation of consumption. On the other hand, a little attention in the early stages, and before sympathetic action sets in, would set all right. The first indication to be fulfilled is to invite action to the surface by friction and counter-irritants. The following liniment may be applied to the feet and throat:—

Olive oil, ...	4 ounces.
Oil of cedar, ...	1 ounce.
Liquid ammonia, ...	half an ounce.

Rub the mixture in well; then give

Gruel, ...	1 quart.
Powdered licorice, ...	1 ounce.
Composition, ...	half a tea-spoonful.

Give this at a dose, and repeat two or three times during the twenty-four hours. A drink of any warm aromatic tea, *such as pennyroyal, hyssop, catnip or aniseed will have a good effect.* The diet should consist of scalded meal, boiled carrots, flaxseed, or any substance that is light and easy of digestion. Should the discharge increase and the eyelids swell, recourse must be had to vapor, which may be raised by pouring vinegar on a hot brick; the latter held, with a pair of tongs, beneath the animal's nose, at the same time covering the head with a blanket. A small quantity of bayberry bark may occasionally be blown up the nostrils from a quill. It is very important, during the treatment, that the animal be in a warm situation, with a good bed of straw to rest on. If the glands under the jaw enlarge, the following mixture should be rubbed about the throat:—

Neat's foot oil, ...	4 ounces.
Hot drops, ...	2 ounces.
Vinegar, ...	1 gill.

If the disease assumes a chronic form, and the animal is evidently losing flesh, then give the following:—

Golden seal, powdered, . . .	1 table-spoonful.
Caraway seeds, " . . .	1 "

Divide into three parts; which may be given daily, (in thin gruel,) until the animal is convalescent.

EPIDEMIC CATARRH.

This often prevails at particular seasons, and spreads over whole districts, sometimes destroying a great number of cattle. It is a disorder whose intensity varies considerably, being sometimes attended with a high grade of fever, at other times quickly followed by general debility.

Treatment.—This requires the same treatment as the last-named disease, but only more thoroughly and perseveringly applied; for every portion of the system seems to be affected, either through sympathetic action or from the absorption of morbid matter. Hence we must aid the vital power to maintain her empire and resist the encroachments on her sanative operations by the use of antispetics and stimulants. The following is a good example: —

Powdered charcoal, ...	1 ounce.
" bayberry bark, ...	half an ounce.
" plurisy root, ...	1 ounce.
Honey, ...	1 table-spoonful.
Thin gruel, ...	1 quart.

MALIGNANT EPIDEMIC, (MURRAIN.)

This disease has been more or less destructive from the time of Pharaoh up to the present period. For information on the origin, progress, and termination of this malignant distemper, the reader is referred to Mr. Youatt's work on cattle.

Treatment. — The indications to be fulfilled are, first, to preserve the system from putrescence, which can be done by the use of the following drink: —

Powdered capsicum, ...	1 tea-spoonful.
" charcoal, ...	2 ounces.
Lime water, ...	4 ounces.
Sulphur, ...	1 tea-spoonful.

Add to the capsicum, charcoal, and sulphur, a small quantity of gruel; lastly, add the lime water. A second and similar dose may be given six hours after the first, provided, however, the symptoms are not so alarming.

The next indication is, to break down the morbid action of the nervous and vascular systems; for which the following may be given freely: —

Thoroughwort tea, ...	2 quarts.
Powdered assafœtida, . . .	2 drachms.

Aid the action of these remedies by the use of one of the following injections: —

Powdered lobelia, ...	2 ounces.
Oil of peppermint, ...	20 drops.
Warm water, ...	2 quarts.

Another.

Infusion of camomile, ...	2 quarts.
Common salt, ...	4 ounces.

In all cases of putrid or malignant fever, efforts should be made to supply the system with caloric, (by the aid of stimulants,) promote the secretions, and rid the system of morbific materials.

DIARRHŒA, (Looseness of the Bowels.)

In the early stages of this disease, it is not always to be checked. It is often a salutary operation of nature to rid the system of morbific materials, and all that we can do with safety is, to sheathe and lubricate the mucous surfaces, in order to protect them from the acrid and stimulating properties of the agents to be removed from the alimentary canal.

When the disease, of which diarrhœa is only a symptom, proceeds from exposure, apply warmth, moisture, friction, and stimulants to the external surface, aided by the following lubricant: —

Powdered slippery elm, ...	1 ounce.
" charcoal, ...	1 table-spoonful.
Boiling water, ...	2 quarts.

Common starch, or flour, may be substituted for slippery elm. The mixture should be given in pint doses, at intervals of two hours. When the fecal discharges appear more natural and less frequent, a tea of raspberry leaves or bayberry bark will complete the cure.

When the disease assumes a chronic form, and the animal

loses flesh, the following tonic, stimulating, astringent drink is recommended: —

Infusion of camomile,	. . . . . .	1 quart.
Powdered caraway seeds,	. . . . .	1 ounce.
Bayberry, powdered,	. . . . . .	half an ounce.

Mix for one dose.

Remarks. — In the treatment of this disease, it is necessary for the farmer to know, that through the instrumentality of the nervous structure, there is constantly a sympathy kept up between the different parts of the animal; whenever any part is affected, the corresponding part feels the influence. Thus the external surface is opposed to the internal, so that, if the function of the former be diminished, or excessive, or suspended, that of the latter will soon become deranged; and the restoration of the lost function is the only true way to effect a cure. For example, if an animal be suffered to feed in wet lands, the feet and external surface become cold; and hence diarrhœa, catarrh, garget, dysentery, &c. If the circulation of the blood is obstructed by exposure, we should restore the lost function by rubbing the surface, and by the application of warmth and moisture. If the animal is in poor condition, and there is not enough vitality to equalize the circulation, give warm anti-spasmodics. (See APPENDIX.) In cases where diarrhœa results from a want of power in the digestive organs to assimilate the food, the latter acts on the mucous surfaces as a mechanical irritant, producing inflammation, &c. Inflammation is the concentration of the available vital force too much upon a small region of the body, and it is invited there by irritation. Now, instead of the popular error, — bleeding and purging, — the most rational way to proceed is, to remove the cause of irritation, (no matter whether the stomach or bowels are involved,) and invite the blood to the surface by means already alluded to, and distribute it over the general system, so that it will not be in excess any where. There is generally but little difficulty in producing an equilibrium of action; the great point is to sustain it. When the blood accumulates in a part, as in inflammation of the bowels, the sensibility of the part is so highly exalted that the least irritation causes a relapse; therefore the general treatment must not be abandoned too early.

DYSENTERY.

The disease is generally ushered in with some degree of fever; as, trembling, hot and cold stages, dryness of the mouth, loss of appetite, general prostration, drooping of the head and ears, heaving of the flanks; there are frequent stools, yet these seldom consist of natural excrement, but are of a viscid, mucous character; the animal is evidently in pain during these discharges, and sometimes the fundament appears excoriated.

Causes. — The cause of this complaint appears to be, generally, exposure. Dr. White says, "Almost all the diseases of cattle arise either from exposure to wet or cold weather, from their food being of a bad quality, or deficient in quantity, or from the animal being changed too suddenly from poor, unwholesome keep to rich pasture. It is necessary to observe, also, that the animal is more liable to be injured by exposure to wet and cold, when previously enfeebled by bad keep, old age, or any other cause; and particularly when brought from a mild into a cold situation. I have scarcelv met with a disease that is not attributable to a chill."

Treatment. — This must be much the same as in diarrhœa — sheathing the mucous membrane, and inviting action to the surface. The animal must be warmly housed, well littered, and the extremities clothed with flannel bandages. The diet must consist of flour gruel, scalded meal. Raspberry tea will be the most suitable drink. Much can be done by good nursing. Mr. Ellman says, "If any of my cattle get into a low weak state, I generally recommend nursing, which, in most cases, is much better than a doctor; [meaning some of the poor specimens always to be found in large cities;] having often seen the beast much weakened, and the stomach relaxed, by throwing in a quantity of medicine injudiciously, and the animal lost; when, with good nursing, in all probability, it might have been otherwise."

SCOURING ROT.

Cause. — Any thing that can reduce the vital energies.

Symptoms. — A gradual loss of flesh, although the animal often feeds well and ruminates. The excrements are of a dark color, frothy, and fetid, and, in the latter stages, appear to be only half digested. There are many symptoms and different degrees of intensity, during the progress of this disease, which indicate the amount of destruction going on; yet the author considers them unimportant in a practical point of view, at least as far as the treatment is concerned; for the disease is so analogous to dysentery, that the same indications are to be fulfilled in both; more care, however, should be taken to prevent and subdue mortification.

In addition to the treatment recommended in article *Malignant Epidemic*, the following injection may be substituted for the one prescribed under that head: —

Powdered charcoal, ...	a tea-cupful.
Common salt, ...	2 ounces.
Pyroligneous acid,*	half a wine-glass.
Warm water, ...	2 quarts.

Throw one quart of the above into the rectum, and the remainder six hours after the first.

* Vinegar obtained from wood.

DISEASE OF THE EAR.

Diseases of the ear are very rare in cattle, yet, as simple inflammatory action does now and then occur, it is well that the farmer should be able to recognize and treat it.

Symptoms.—An unnatural heat and tenderness about the base of the ear, and the animal carries the head on one side.

Cure.—Fomentations of marshmallows; a light diet of scalded shorts; an occasional drink of thoroughwort tea These with a little rest, in a comfortable barn, will perfect the cure.

Remarks.—If any irritating substance is suspected to have fallen into the ear, efforts must be made to remove it: if it cannot be got at, a small quantity of olive oil may be poured into the cavity; then, by rotating the head, with the affected ear downwards, the substances will often pass out.

SEROUS MEMBRANES.

These membranes derive their name from the serous or watery fluid they secrete, by which their surface is constantly moistened. They are to be found in the three cavities of the chest; namely, one on each side, containing the right and left lung, and the intermediate cavity, occupied by the heart. The portion of the membrane lining the lungs is named the *pleura*, and that lining and covering the heart is called the *pericardium.* The membrane lining the abdomen is named the *peritoneum.* The ventricles of the brain are also lined by this membrane. The serous membranes, after lining their respective cavities, are extended still farther, by being reflected back upon the organs enclosed in their cavities; hence, if it were possible to dissect these membranes from off the parts which they invest, they would have the appearance of a sac without an opening. In the natural state, these membranes are exceedingly thin and transparent; but they become thickened by disease, and lose their transparency. The excessive discharge of fluids into cavities lined by these membranes constitutes the different forms of dropsy, on which we shall now treat.

DROPSY.

This disease consists in the accumulation of fluid in a cavity of the body, as the abdomen or belly, the chest, and ventricles of the brain, or in the cellular membrane under the skin. As the treatment of the several forms of dropsy requires that the same indications shall be fulfilled, — viz., to equalize the circulation, invite action to the surface, promote absorption, and invigorate the general system, — so it matters but little whether the effusion takes place under the skin, producing anasarca, or within the chest or abdomen. The popular treatment, which comprehends blood-letting, physicking, and the use of powerful diuretics, has proved notoriously unsuccessful. Blood-letting is charged as one of the direct causes of dropsy: how then can it be expected that a system that will produce this form of disease can ever cure it? In reference to physicking, if the bowels are forced to remove the excess of fluids in a short time, they become much exhausted, lose their tone, and do not recover their healthy power for some time. Dr. Curtis says, "May we not give diuretics and drastic cathartics in dropsy? I answer, if you do, and carry off the fluids of the body in those directions, as you sometimes may, you have not always removed the cause of the disease, which was the closing of the surface or stoppage of some natural secretion, while you have rendered the patient liable to other forms of disease, quite as much to be dreaded as the dropsy which was exchanged for it." Mild diuretic medicines may, however, be given, provided attention be paid at the same time to the lungs and external surface. The kidneys, lungs, and external surface constitute the great outlets through which the excess of fluids finds egress; and if one of these functions be excited to dislodge an accumulation of fluid, without the coöperation of the rest, the excessive action is sure to injure the organ; hence it is an injurious practice, and ought to be rejected.

Causes.—Dropsy will occasionally be produced by the sudden stopping of any evacuation; for example, if a diarrhœa be checked too suddenly, it frequently results in dropsy of the belly. In pleurisy, and when blood-letting has been practised to any extent, dropsy of the chest will be the consequence. Exposure, poor diet, diseases of the liver and spleen, want of exercise, and poisonous medicines are among the general causes of dropsy.

Treatment.—It is a law of the animal economy that all fluids are determined to those surfaces from which they can most readily escape. Now, instead of cramming down nauseous and poisonous drugs, with a view of carrying off the fluid by the kidneys, we should restore the lost function of the external exhalents, by warmth, moisture, friction, and the application of stimulating embrocations to the general surface. The following embrocation may be applied to the spine, ears, belly, and legs:—

Oil of cedar, ...	1 ounce.
Oil of juniper, ...	1 ounce.
Soft soap, ...	1 pound.

A portion of the above should be rubbed in twice a day.

The best medicine is the following: —

Powdered mandrake, ...	1 ounce.
" lobelia, ...	1 ounce.
Poplar bark, ...	2 ounces.
Lemon balm, ...	4 ounces.
Boiling water, ...	3 quarts.

Let the whole stand in a covered vessel for an hour; then strain, and add a gill of honey. Give half a pint every third hour. If the animal be in poor condition, the diet must be nourishing and easy of digestion. Flour gruel and scalded meal will be the most appropriate. A drink made by steeping cleavers, or hyssop, in boiling water may be given at discretion.

If there is not sufficient vitality in the system to equalize the circulation, (which may be known by the surface and extremities still continuing cold,) the following drink will be found efficacious: —

Hyssop tea, ...	2 quarts.
Powdered cayenne, (African,) .	1 tea-spoonful.
" licorice, ...	1 ounce.

Mix. To be given at a dose, and repeated if necessary. Should inflammatory symptoms make their appearance, omit the cayenne, and substitute the same quantity of cream of tartar.

The treatment of all the different forms of dropsy is upon the plan here laid down. They are one and the same disease, only located in different parts; and from predisposing causes the fluid is sometimes found in the thorax, at others in the abdomen. Whenever costiveness occurs in dropsy, the following laxative may be given: —

Wormwood, ...	2 ounces.
Boiling water, ...	2 quarts

Set them over the fire, and let them boil for a few moments; then add two ounces of castile soap and a gill of molasses or honey. The whole to be given at one dose.

The operation of tapping has been performed, but with very little success; for, unless the function of the skin be restored, the water will again accumulate. If, however, the disease shall be treated according to the principles here laid down, there is no good reason why the operation should not prove successful. It may be performed for dropsy of the belly in the following manner: Take a common trocar and canula, and after pinching upwards a fold of the skin, about three inches from the line, (*linea alba,*) or centre of the belly, and about seven from the udder, push the trocar through the skin, muscles, &c., into the abdominal cavity; withdraw the trocar, and the water will flow. The operation is usually performed on the right side, taking care, however, not to wound the milk vein, or artery.

HOOVE, OR "BLASTING."

WHEN cattle or sheep are first turned into luxuriant pasture, after being poorly fed, or laboring under any derangement of the digestive organs, they are apt to be hoven, blown, or blasted.

Treatment. — Should the symptoms be very alarming, a flexible tube may be passed down the gullet. This will generally allow a portion of gas to escape, and thus afford temporary relief, until more efficient means are resorted to. These consist in arousing the digestive organs to action, by the following stimulant and carminative drink: —

Cardamom seeds, ...	1 ounce.
Fennel seeds, ...	1 ounce.
Powdered charcoal, . . .	1 table-spoonful.
Boiling water, ...	2 quarts.

Let the mixture stand until sufficiently cool; then strain, and administer in pint doses, every ten minutes.

The following clyster should be given: —

Powdered lobelia, ...	2 ounces.
" charcoal, ...	6 ounces.
Common salt, ...	1 table-spoonful.
Boiling water, ...	2 quarts.

When cool, strain, and inject.

If the animal is only blasted in a moderate degree, this treatment will generally prove successful. Some practitioners recommend puncturing the rumen or paunch; but there is always great danger attending it, and at best it is only a palliative: the process of fermentation will continue while the materials still remain in the paunch. Some cattle doctors make a large incision into the paunch, and shovel out the contents with the hand; but the remedy is quite as bad as the disease. For example, Mr. Youatt tells us that "a cow had eaten a large quantity of food, and was hoven. A neighbor, who was supposed to know a great deal about cattle, made an incision into the paunch; the gas escaped, a great portion of the food was removed with the hand, and the animal appeared to be considerably relieved; but rumination did not return. On the following day, the animal was dull; she refused her food, but was eager to drink. She became worse and worse, and on the sixth day she died."

In all dangerous cases of hoove, we must not forget that our remedies may be aided by the external application of warmth and moisture; flannels wrung out in hot water should be secured to the belly; at the same time, the legs and brisket should be rubbed with tincture of assafœtida. These remedies must be repeated until the animal is relieved. Steady and long-continued perseverance in rubbing the abdomen often succeeds in liberating the gas. If the animal recovers, he should be fed, very sparingly, on scalded food, consisting of equal parts of meal and shorts, with the addition of a few grains of caraway seeds. A drink composed of the following ingredients will aid in rapidly restoring the animal to health: —

Marshmallows, ...	2 ounces.
Linseed, ...	1 ounce.
Boiling water, ...	2 quarts.

Set the mixture near the fire, and allow it to macerate for a short time; after straining through a sieve or coarse cloth, it may be given and repeated at discretion.

Remarks. — As prevention is much more convenient and less expensive than the fashionable system of making a chemical laboratory of the poor brute's stomach, the author would remind owners of stock that the practice of turning the latter into green, succulent pasture when the ground is damp, or permitting them to remain exposed to the night air, is among the direct causes of hoove. The ox and many other animals are governed by the same laws of nature to which man owes allegiance, and any departure from the legitimate teachings, as they are fundamentally ingrafted in the animate kingdom by the Omnipotent Creator, is sure to subject us to the penalty. We are told that, during the night, noxious gases and poisonous miasmata emanate from the soil, and that plants throw off excrementitious matters, which assume a gaseous form, and are more or less destructive. Now, these animals have no better powers of resisting the encroachments on their organization (through the agency of these deleterious gases) than we have; they must have atmospheric air to vitalize the blood; any impurity in the air they breathe must impair their health. Still, however, the powers of resistance are greater in some than in others; this explains the reason why all do not suffer. Sometimes, the gases are not in sufficient quantities to produce instant death, but only derange the general health; yet if an animal be turned into a pasture, the herbage and soil of which give out an excess of nitrogen and carbonic acid, the animal will die; just as a man will, if you lower him into a well abounding in either of these destructive agents. From these brief remarks, the farmer will see the importance of housing domestic animals at night.

JOINT MURRAIN.

This malady, in its early stages, assumes different forms; sometimes making its appearance under a high grade of vital action, commonly called inflammatory fever, and known by the red appearance of the sclerotica, (white of the eye,) hurried breathing, expanded nostrils, hot tongue, and dry muzzle, pulse full and bounding, manifestations of pain, &c. &c. Different animals show, according to local or constitutional peculiarities, different symptoms.

This disease, in consequence of its assuming different forms during its progress, has a host of names applied to it, which rather embarrass than assist the farmer. We admit that there are numerous tissues to be obstructed; and if the disease were named from the tissue, it would have as many names as there are tissues. If it were named from the location, which often happens, then we get as many names as there are locations; for example, horn ail, black leg, quarter evil, joint murrain, foot rot, &c. In the above disease, the whole system partakes more or less of constitutional disturbance; therefore it is of no use, except when we want to avail ourselves of local applications, to decide what particular muscle, blood-vessel, or nerve is involved, seeing that the only rational treatment consists in acting on all the nerves, blood-vessels, and muscles, and that this can only be accomplished through the healthy operations of nature's secreting and excreting processes. The indications of cure, according to the reformed principles, are, to relax spasm, as in locked-jaw, stoppages of the bladder or intestines, obstructed surfaces, &c.; to contract and strengthen weak and relaxed organs, as in general or local debility, diarrhœa, scouring, lampas, &c.; to stimulate inactive parts, as in black leg, joint murrain, quarter ill, foot rot; to equalize the circulation, and distribute the blood to the external surface and extremities, as in congestions; to furnish the animal with sufficient nutriment for its growth and development. No matter what the nature of disease may be, the treatment should be conducted on these principles.

The farmer will overcome a host of obstacles, that might otherwise fall in his way, in the treatment of joint murrain, when he learns that this malady, together with black leg, quarter ill or evil, black quarter, and dry gangrene are all analogous: by the different names are meant their grades. In the early or mild forms, it consists of congestion in the veins or venous radicles, and effusions into the cellular tissue. When chemical action overpowers the vital, decomposition sets in; it then assumes a putrid type; mortification, or a destruction of organic integrity, is the result.

Causes. — Its proximate causes exist in any thing that can for a time interrupt the free and full play of any part of the vital machinery. Its direct cause may be found in over-feeding, miasma, exposure, poisonous plants, poor diet, &c. The milk of diseased cows is a frequent cause of black leg in young calves. The reason why the disease is more likely to manifest itself in the legs is, because they are more exposed, by the feet coming in contact with damp ground, and because the blood has a kind of up-hill work to perform.

Treatment. — In the early stages of joint murrain and its kindred maladies, if inflammatory fever is present, the first aud most important step is to relax the external surface, as directed in article *Pneumonia*, p. 107. Should the animal be in a situation where it is not convenient to do so, give the following anti-spasmodic: —

Thoroughwort, ...	1 ounce.
Lemon balm, ...	2 ounces.
Garlic, bruised, ...	a few kernels.
Boiling water, ...	3 quarts.

Allow the infusion to stand until cool; then strain, and give it a dose.

If the bowels are constipated, inject the following: —

Soft soap, ...	half a pint.
Warm water, ...	2 quarts.

Rub the joints with the following embrocation:—

Oil of cedar,	. . . .	equal parts.
Fir balsam,	. . . .	

Keep the animal on warm, bland teas, such as catnip, pennyroyal, lemon balm, and a light diet of powdered slippery elm gruel.

BLACK QUARTER.

Symptoms.—Rapid decomposition, known by the pain which the slightest pressure gives the animal. Carbonic acid gas is evolved from the semi-putrid state of the system, which finds its way into the cellular tissue, beneath the skin. A crackling noise can then be heard and felt by pressing the finger on the hide.

Causes.—Among the chief causes are the blood-letting and scouring systems recommended by writers on cattle doctoring. In the inflammatory stage, we are told, "The first and most important step is copious bleeding. As much blood must be taken as the animal will bear to lose; and the stream must flow on until the beast staggers or threatens to fall. Here, more than in any other disease, there must be no foolish directions about quantities. [*The heroic practice!*] As much blood must be taken away as can be got; for it is only by the bold and persevering use of the lancet that a malady can be subdued that runs its course so rapidly." (See Youatt, p. 359.) From these directions we are led to suppose that there are some hopes of bleeding the animal to life; for the author above quoted seems to entertain no apprehension of bleeding the animal to death. Mr. Percival and other veterinary writers inform us, that "an animal will lose about one fifteenth part of its weight of blood before it dies; though a less quantity may so far debilitate the vital powers, as to be, though less suddenly equally fatal." The latter portion of the sentence means simply this; that if the bleeding does not give the animal its quietus on the spot, it will produce black quarter, gangrene, &c., which will be "equally fatal." In the latter stages of the disease now under consideration, and, indeed, in dry gangrene, there is a tendency to the complete destruction of life to the parts involved: hence our remedies should be in harmony with the vital operations. We should relax, stimulate, and cleanse the whole system, and arouse every part to healthy action, by the aid of vapor, injections, stimulating applications, poultices of charcoal and capsicum, to parts where there is danger of rapid mortification; lastly, stimulating drinks to vitalize the blood, which only requires distribution, instead of abstraction.

In reference to the scouring system, (purging,) as a cause of mortification, we leave the reader to form his own views, after reading the following: "After abstracting as much blood as can be got away, purging must immediately follow. A pound and a half of Epsom salts dissolved in water or gruel, and poured down the throat as gently as possible, should be our first dose. If this does not operate in the course of six hours, another pound should be given; and after that, half pound doses every six hours until the effect is produced"!! — *Youatt*, p. 359.

Treatment. — As the natural tendency of these different maladies is the complete destruction of life to all parts of the organization, efforts must be made to depurate the whole animal, and arouse every part to healthy action in the manner recommended under article *Joint Murrain.* Antiseptics may be freely used in the following form: —

Powdered bayberry bark, ...	2 ounces.
" charcoal, ...	6 ounces.
" cayenne, ...	1 tea-spoonful.
" slippery elm, ...	1 ounce.

Add boiling water sufficient to make it of the consistence of thin gruel.

All sores and foul ulcers may be washed with

Pyroligneous acid,	. . . .	1 ounce.
Water,	. . . .	1 gill.

Another.

Chloride of lime,	. . . .	1 ounce.
Water,	. . . .	1 pint.

Another.

Chloride of soda,	. . . .	1 ounce.
Water,	. . . .	6 ounces.

The affected parts should be often bathed with one of these washes. If the disease is not arrested by these means, repeat them, and put the animal on a diet of flour gruel.

OPEN JOINT.

Joints are liable to external injury from wounds or bruises, and, although a joint may not be open in the first instance, subsequent sloughing may expose its cavity. The ordinary effects of disease in membranes covering joints are, a profuse discharge of joint oil, (*synovia,*) and a thickening of the synovial membrane. Sometimes the joint is cemented together; it is then termed anchylosis.

Treatment. — The first object is, to promote adhesion, by bringing the edges of the wound together, and confining them in contact by stitches. A pledget of lint or linen, previously moistened with tincture of myrrh, should then be bound on with a bandage forming a figure 8 around the joint. If the parts feel hot and appear inflamed, apply a bandage, which may be kept constantly wet with cold water. If adhesion of the parts does not take place, apply the following: —

Powdered bayberry bark,	. . . . .	1 ounce.

Fir balsam, sufficient to form a thick, tenacious mass, which may be spread thickly over the wound; lastly, a bandage. Should a fetid discharge take place, poultice with

Powdered charcoal,	. . . . . .	equal parts.
" bayberry,	. . . . . .	

In cases where the nature of the injury will not admit of the wounded edges being kept in contact, and a large surface is exposed, we must promote granulation by keeping the parts clean, and by the daily application of fir balsam. Unhealthy granulations may be kept down by touching them with burnt alum, or sprinkling on their surface powdered bloodroot. The author has treated several cases, in which there was no hope of healing by the first intention, by the daily use of tincture of capsicum, together with tonic, stimulating, astringent, antiseptic poultices and fomentations, as the case seemed to require, and they always terminated favorably. In all cases of injury to joints, rest and a light diet are indispensable.

SWELLINGS OF JOINTS.

Swellings frequently arise from bruises and strains; they are sometimes, however, connected with a rheumatic affection, caused by cold, exposure to rain, or turning an animal into wet pasture lands after active exercise. In the acute stage, known by tenderness, unnatural heat, and lameness, the animal should be put on a light diet of scalded shorts, &c.; the parts to be frequently bathed with cold water; and, if practicable, a bandage may be passed around the limb, and kept moist with the same. If the part still continues painful, take four ounces of arnica flowers, moisten them with boiling water, when cool, bind them around the part, and let them remain twenty-four hours. This seldom fails. On the other hand, should the parts be in a chronic state, which may be recognized by inactivity, coldness, &c., then the following embrocation will restore the lost tone: —

Oil of wormwood, ...	1 ounce.
" " cedar, ...	1 ounce.
Hot drops, ...	4 ounces.
Vinegar, ...	1 pint.

Mix, and rub the part faithfully night and morning. Friction with the hand or a brush will materially assist to cure. In all cases where suppuration has commenced, and matter can be distinctly felt, the sooner the following poultice shall be applied, the better: —

Powdered slippery elm, . .	equal parts.
" linseed, ...	

Boiling water sufficient to moisten; then add a wine-glass of vinegar.

To be renewed every twelve hours, until the matter escapes.

SPRAIN OF THE FETLOCK.

Sprain, or *strain*, as it is commonly termed, sometimes arises from violent exertions; at other times, by the animal unexpectedly treading on some uneven surface.

Treatment. — First wash the foot clean, then carefully examine the cleft, and remove any substance that may have lodged there. A cotton bandage folded around the claws and continued above the fetlock, kept wet with the following lotion, will speedily reduce any excess of inflammatory action that may exist: —

Acetic acid, ...	1 ounce.
Water, ...	1 pint.

Another.

Vinegar, ...	1 pint.
Water, ...	3 pints.

STRAIN OF THE HIP.

This may sometimes occur in working oxen. Rest is the principal remedy. The part may, however, be bathed daily with the following: —

Wormwood, ...	4 ounces.
Scalding vinegar, ...	2 quarts.

The liquor must be applied cold.

Strain of the knees or *shoulder* may be treated in the same manner as above.

FOUL IN THE FOOT.

A great deal of learned nonsense has been written on this subject, which only serves to plunge the farmer into a labyrinth from which there is no escape. The author will not trespass on the reader's patience so much as to transcribe different authors' opinions in relation to the nature of the disease and its treatment, but will proceed at once to point out a common-sense explanation of its cause, and the proper mode of treating it.

The disease is analogous to foot rot in sheep, and is the consequence of feeding in wet pastures, or suffering the animals to wallow in filth. A large quantity of morbific or excrementitious matter is thrown off from the system through the surfaces between the cleft. Now, should those surfaces be obstructed by filth, or contracted by cold, the delicate mouths of these excrementitious vessels, or outlets, are unable to rid the parts of their morbid accumulations: these vessels become distended beyond their usual capacity, communicate with each other, and, when no longer able to contain this mass of useless material, an artificial drain, in the form of "foot rot," is established, by which simple method the parts recover their reciprocal equilibrium. In this case, as in diarrhœa, we recognize a simple and sanative operation of nature's law, which, if aided, will generally prove beneficial.

That "foul in the foot" is caused by the sudden stoppage of some natural evacuation is evident from the following facts: First, the disease is most prevalent in cold, low, marshy countries, where the foot is kept constantly moist. Secondly, the disease is neither contagious nor epidemic. (See *Journal de Méd. Vét. et comparée,* 1826, p. 319.)

Treatment. — In all cases of obstruction to the depurating apparatus, there is a loss of equilibrium between secretion and excretion. The first indication is, to restore the lost function. Previously, however, to doing so, the animal must be removed to a dry situation. The cause once removed, the cure is easy, provided we merely assist nature and follow her teachings. As warmth and moisture are known to relax all animal fibre, the part should be relaxed, warmed, and cleansed, first by warm water and soap, lastly by poultice; at the same time bearing in mind that the object is not to produce or invite suppuration, (formation of matter,) but only to liberate the excess of morbid materials that may already be present: as soon as this is accomplished, the poultice should be discontinued.

Poultice for Foul Feet.

Roots of marshmallows, bruised, .	half a pound.
Powdered charcoal, ...	a handful.
" lobelia, ...	a few ounces.
Meal.	a tea-cupful.

Boiling water sufficient to soften the mass

Another.

Powdered lobelia, ...	equal parts.
Slippery elm, ...	
Pond lily, bruised, ...	

Mix with boiling water. Put the ingredients into a bag and secure it above the fetlock.

Give the animal the following at a dose:—

Flowers of sulphur, ...	half an ounce.
Powdered sassafras bark, . . .	1 ounce.
Burdock, (any part of the plant,) .	2 ounces.

The above to be steeped in one quart of boiling water When cool, strain. All that is now needed is to keep the part cleansed, and at rest. If a fetid smell still remains, wet the cleft, morning and evening, with

Chloride of soda, ...	1 ounce.
Water, ...	6 ounces.

Mix.

Another.

Pyroligneous acid, ...	2 ounces.
Water, ...	a pint.

Mix.

Another.

Common salt, ...	1 table-spoonful.
Vinegar, ...	a wine-glass.
Water, ...	1 quart.

Whenever any fungous excrescence makes its appearance between the claws, apply powdered bloodroot c burnt alum.

RED WATER.

This affection takes its name from the high color of the urine. It is not, strictly speaking, a disease, but only a symptom of derangement, caused by high feeding or the suppression of some natural discharge. If, for example, the skin be obstructed, then the insensible perspiration and excrementitious matter, which should pass through this great outlet, find some other mode of egress; either the lungs or kidneys have to perform the extra work. If the lot falls on the latter, and they are not in a physiological state, they give evidence of febrile or inflammatory action (caused by the irritating, acrid character of their secretion) in the form of high-colored urine. In all cases of derangement in the digestive apparatus, liver included, both in man and oxen, the urine is generally high colored; and the use of diuretic medicines is objectionable, for, at best, it would only be treating symptoms. We lay it down as a fundamental principle, that those who treat symptoms alone never cure disease, for the animal often dies a victim to the treatment, instead of the malady.

Whenever an animal is in a state of plethora, and the usual amount of morbific matter cannot find egress, some portion of it is reabsorbed, producing a deleterious effect: the urine will then be high colored, plainly demonstrating that nature is making an effort to rid the system of useless material, and will do so unless interfered with by the use of means opposed to the cure, such as blood-letting, physicking, and diuretics.

The urine will appear high colored, and approach a red hue, in many cows after calving, in inflammation of the womb, gastric fever, puerperal fever, fevers generally, inflammation of the kidneys, indigestion; in short, many forms of acute disease are accompanied by high-colored urine.

The treatment, like that of any other form of derangement, must be general. Excite all parts of the system to healthy action. If the bowels are constipated, give the following:

Golden seal, ...	1 table-spoonful.
Thoroughwort tea, . . .	2 quarts.

To be given at a dose. Scalded shorts will be the most suitable food, if any is required; but, generally, abstinence is necessary, especially if the animal be fat. If the surface and extremities are cold, give an infusion of pennyroyal, catnip, sage, or hyssop; and rub the belly and legs with

Hot vinegar, ...	1 quart.
Powdered lobelia or cayenne, . .	1 ounce.

If the kidneys are inflamed,—which may be known by tenderness in the region of the loins, and by the animal standing with the legs widely separated,—the urine being of a dark red color, then, in addition to the application of stimulating liniment to the belly and legs, a poultice may be placed over the kidneys.

Poultice for inflamed Kidneys.

Slippery elm, ...	8 ounces.
Lobelia, ...	4 ounces.
Boiling water sufficient.	

Another.

Linseed, ...	equal parts.
Marshmallows, ...	
Boiling water sufficient.	

Lay the poultice on the loins, pass a cloth over it, and secure under the belly.

A drink of marshmallows is the only fluid that can with safety be allowed.

If the horns, ears, and surface are hot, sponge the whole surface with weak lie or saleratus water, and give the following antifebrile drink:—

Lemon balm, ...	2 ounces.
Cream of tartar, ...	1 ounce.
Boiling water, ...	2 quarts.
Honey, ...	1 gill.

When cold, strain, and give a pint every fifteen minutes

If the bowels are constipated, use injections of soap-suds.

Suppose the animal to be in poor condition, hide bound, liver inactive, the excrement of a dark color and fetid odor. Then use

Powdered golden seal, . . .	2 ounces.
" caraways, ...	1 ounce.
" cayenne, ...	1 tea-spoonful.
Poplar bark, or slippery elm, .	2 ounces.

Mix, divide into ten parts, and give one, in thin gruel, three times a day. The animal should be fed on boiled carrots, scalded shorts, into which a few handfuls of meal or flour may be stirred. In short, consider the nature of the case; look beyond the symptoms, ascertain the cause, and, if possible, remove it. An infusion of either of the following articles may be given at discretion: marshmallows, linseed, juniper berries, pond lily roots, poplar bark, or queen of the meadow.

Mr. Cole remarks that "red water is most common in cows of weak constitution, a general relaxation, poor blood, &c."

In such cases, a nutritious diet, cleanliness, good nursing, friction on the surface, comfortable quarters at night, and an occasional tonic will accomplish wonders.

Tonic Mixture.

Powdered golden seal, . . .	1 tea-spoonful.
" balmony, . . .	2 tea-spoonfuls.

Mix the above in shorts or meal. Repeat night and morning until convalescence is established. In cases of great prostration, where it is necessary to act with promptitude, the following infusion may be substituted: —

Thoroughwort, ...	of each, 1 ounce.
Golden seal, ...	
Camomile flowers, ...	
Boiling water, ...	2 quarts.

After standing one hour, strain, and give a pint every four hours

BLACK WATER.

My plan of treatment, in this malady, is similar to that for red water. In both cases, it is indispensable to attend to the general health, to promote the discharge of all the secretions, to remove all obstructions to the full and free play of all parts of the living machinery. The same remedies recommended in the preceding article are equally good in this case, only they must be more perseveringly applied.

THICK URINE.

Whenever the urine is thick and turbid, deficient in quantity, or voided with difficulty, either of the following prescriptions may be administered:—

Juniper berries, ...	2 ounces.
Boiling water, ...	2 quarts.

Strain. Dose, 1 pint every four hours.

Another.

Slippery elm, ...	1 ounce.
Poplar bark, ...	2 ounces.

Make a tea; sweeten with molasses, and give pint doses every four hours.

Another.

Make a tea of cedar or pine boughs, sweeten with honey, and give it at discretion.

RHEUMATISM.

Rheumatism thrives in cold, damp situations, and in wet foggy weather. It is often confined to the membranes of the large joints, and sometimes consists in a deficiency of joint oil, (*synovia.*) It is liable to become chronic, and involve the fibro-muscular tissues. Acute rheumatism is known by the pain and swelling in certain parts. Chronic rheumatism is recognized by coldness, rigidity about the muscles, want of vital action, &c.

When lameness, after a careful examination, cannot be accounted for, and is found to go off after exercise, and return again, it is probably rheumatism.

Treatment of Acute Rheumatism. — Bathe the parts with an infusion of arnica flowers, made thus: —

Arnica flowers, ...	4 ounces.
Boiling water, ...	3 quarts.

When sufficiently cool, it is fit for use.

Give the following: —

Sulphur, ...	2 ounces.
Cream of tartar, ...	3 ounces.
Powdered pleurisy root, ...	1 ounce.
" licorice, ...	2 ounces.
Indian meal, ...	1 pound.

Mix. Give a table-spoonful three times a day in the feed A light diet and rest are indispensable.

Treatment of Chronic Rheumatism. — Put the animal on a generous diet, and give an occasional spoonful of golden seal or balmony in the food, and a drink of sassafras tea. The parts may be rubbed with stimulating liniment, for which, see Appendix

BLAINE.

SOME veterinary writers describe this disease as "a watery tumor, growing at the root of the tongue, and threatening suffocation. The first symptoms are foaming at the mouth, gaping, and lolling out of the tongue."

The disease first originates in the mucous surfaces, which enter into the mouth, throat, and stomach. It partakes somewhat of the character of thrush, and requires nearly the same treatment.

Make an infusion of raspberry leaves, to which add a small quantity of borax or alum. Wash the mouth and tongue with the same by means of a sponge. If there are any large pustules, open them with the point of a penknife. After cleansing them, sprinkle with powdered bayberry bark, or bloodroot. Rid the system of morbid matter by injection and physic, (which see, in APPENDIX.) The following antiseptic drink will then complete the cure: —

Make a tea of raspberry leaves by steeping two ounces in a quart of boiling water; when cool, strain; then add

Powdered charcoal, ...	2 ounces.
" bayberry bark, . .	1 ounce.
Honey, ...	2 table-spoonfuls.

Give a pint every four hours.

The diet should consist of scalded meal, boiled turnips, carrots, &c., to which a small portion of salt may be added. If the glands under the ears and around the throat are sympathetically affected, and swollen, they must be rubbed twice a day with the stimulating liniment. (See APPENDIX.)

The disease is supposed, by some veterinarians, to originate in the tongue, but post mortem examinations lead us to determine otherwise. Mr. Youatt informs us that "post mortem examination shows intense inflammation, or even gangrene, of the tongue, œsophagus, paunch, and fourth stomach. The food in the paunch has a most offensive smell, and that in the manyplus is hard and dry. Inflammation reaches to the small intestines, which are covered with red and black patches in the cœcum, colon, and rectum."

THRUSH.

Thrush, and all eruptive diseases of the throat and internal surface, are treated in the same manner as laid down in Blaine.

BLACK TONGUE.

Black Tongue appears when the system is deprived of vital force, as in the last stages of blaine, &c. The indications to be fulfilled are the same as in blaine, but applied with more perseverance.

INFLAMMATION OF THE THROAT AND ITS APPENDAGES.*

In many cases, if attended to immediately, nothing more will be necessary than confining the animal to a light diet, with frequent drinks of linseed tea, warmth and moisture applied locally in the form of a slippery elm poultice, which may be kept in close contact with the throat by securing it to the horns. But, in very severe attacks, mullein leaves steeped in vinegar and applied to the parts, with an occasional stimulating injection, (see Appendix,) together with a gruel diet, are the only means of relief.

* This includes the larynx, pharynx, and trachea.

BRONCHITIS.

Bronchitis consists in a thickening of the fibrous and mucous surfaces of the trachea, and generally results from maltreated hoose or catarrh.

Symptoms. — A dry, husky, wheezing cough laborious breathing, hot breath, and dry tongue.

Treatment. — Warm poultices of slippery elm or flaxseed, on the surface of which sprinkle powdered lobelia. Apply them to the throat moderately warm; if they are too hot they will prove injurious. In the first place administer the following drink: —

Powdered licorice, ...	1 ounce.
" elecampane, ...	half an ounce.
Slippery elm, ...	1 ounce.

Boiling water sufficient to make it of the consistence of thin gruel.

If there is great difficulty of breathing, add half a tea-spoon of lobelia to the above, and repeat the dose night and morning. Linseed or marshmallow tea is a valuable auxiliary in the treatment of this disease. The animal should be comfortably housed, and the legs kept warm by friction with coarse straw.

INFLAMMATION OF GLANDS.

There are numerous glandular bodies distributed over the animal structure. Those to which the reader's attention is called are, first, the parotid, situated beneath the ear; secondly, the sub-lingual, beneath the tongue; lastly, the submaxillary, situated iust within the angle of the jaw. Thev are organized similarly to other glands, as the kidneys, &c., possessing arteries, veins, lymphatics, &c., which terminate in a common duct. They have also a ramification of nerves, and the body of the gland has its own system of arterial vessels and absorbents, which are enclosed by a serous membrane. They produce a copious discharge of fluid, called saliva. Its use is to lubricate the mouth, thereby preventing friction; also to lubricate the food, and assist digestion.

Inflammation of either of these glands may be known by the heat, tenderness, enlargement, and difficulty of swallowing. They are usually sympathetically affected, as in hoose, catarrh, influenza, &c., and generally resume their natural state when these maladies disappear.

Treatment.—In the inflammatory stage, warm teas of marshmallows, or slippery elm, and poultices of the same, are the best means yet known to reduce it; they relax constricted or obstructed organs, and by being directly applied to the parts affected, the more speedily and effectually is the object accomplished. Two or three applications of some relaxing poultice will be all that is needed; after which, apply

Olive oil, or goose grease, . . .	1 gill.
Spirits of camphor, ...	1 ounce.
Oil of cedar, ...	1 ounce.
Vinegar, ...	half a gill.

Mix.

Another.

Pyroligneous acid, ...	2 ounces.
Beef's gall, ...	1 gill.
Cayenne, ...	1 tea-spoonful.

To be rubbed around the throat as occasion may require. All hard or indigestible food will be injurious.

LOSS OF CUD.

Loss of Cud is a species of indigestion, and may be brought on by the animal's eating greedily of some food to which it has been unaccustomed. Loss of cud and loss of appetite are synonymous.

Compound for Loss of Cud.

Golden seal, powdered, ...	1 ounce.
Caraway, "	2 ounces.
Cream of tartar, ...	half an ounce.
Powdered poplar bark, ...	2 ounces.

Mix. Divide into six powders, and give one every four hours in a sufficient quantity of camomile tea.

COLIC.

Colic is occasioned by a want of physiological power in the organs of digestion, so that the food, instead of undergoing a chemico-vital process, runs into fermentation, by which process carbonic acid gas is evolved.

Symptoms. — The animal is evidently in pain, and appears very restless; it occasionally turns its head, with an anxious gaze, to the left side, which seems to be distended more than the right; there is an occasional discharge of gas from the mouth and anus.

Treatment. — Give the following carminative: —

Powdered aniseed, ...	half a tea-spoonful.
" cinnamon, . . .	" "

To be given in a quart of spearmint tea, and repeated if necessary.

Another.

Powdered assafœtida, ...	half a tea-spoon.
Thin gruel of slippery elm, . . .	2 quarts.
Oil of aniseed, ...	20 drops.

To be given at a dose.

If the animal suffers much pain, apply fomentations to the belly, and give the following injection: —

Powdered ginger, ...	half an ounce.
Common salt, ...	1 table-spoonful.
Hot water, ...	1 gallon.

SPASMODIC COLIC.

This affection may be treated in the same manner as flatulent colic, aided by warmth and moisture externally. The author has in many cases cured animals of spasmodic colic with a little peppermint tea, brisk friction upon the stomach and bowels, and an injection of warm water; whereas, had the animals been compelled to swallow the usual amount of gin, saleratus, castor oil, salts, and other nauseous, useless drugs, they would probably have died. The reader, especially if he is an advocate of the popular poisoning and blood-letting system, may ask, What good can a little simple peppermint tea accomplish? We answer, Nature delights in simples, and in all her operations invites us to follow her example. The fact is, warm peppermint tea, although in the estimation of the learned it is not entitled to any confidence as a therapeutic agent, yet is an efficient anti-spasmodic in the hands of reformers and common-sense farmers. It is evident that if any changes are made in the symptoms, they ought to be for the better; yet under the heroic practice they often grow worse

---

CONSTIPATION.

In constipation there is a retention of the excrement, which becomes dry and hard. It may arise from derangement of the liver and other parts of the digestive apparatus: at other times, there is a loss of equilibrium between the mucous and external surface, the secretion of the former being deficient, and the external surface throwing off too much moisture in the form of perspiration. In short, constipation, in nine cases out of ten, is only a symptom of a more serious disorder in some important function. The use of powerful purges is at all times attended with danger, and in very many cases they fall short of accomplishing the object. Mr. Youatt tells us that "a heifer had been feverish, and had refused all food during five days; and four pounds of Epsom salts, and the same quantity of treacle, and three fourths of a pint of castor oil, and numerous injections, had been administered before any purgative effect could be produced." Several cases have come under the author's notice where large doses of aloes, salts and castor oil had been given without producing the least effect on the bowels, until within a few minutes of the death of the animal. If the animal ever recovers from the dangerous effects resulting from powerful purges, it is evident that the delicate membranes lining the alimentary canal must lose their energy and become torpid. All mechanical irritants — for purges are of that class — divert the fluids of the body from the surface and kidneys, producing watery discharges from the bowels. This may be exemplified by a person taking a pinch of snuff; the irritating article comes in contact with the mucous surfaces: they endeavor to wash off the offending matter by secreting a quantity of fluid; this, together with what is forced through the membranes in the act of sneezing, generally accomplishes the purpose. A constant repetition of the vile habit renders the parts less capable of self-defence; they become torpid, and lose their natural power of resisting encroachments; finally, the altered voice denotes the havoc made on the mucous membrane. This explains the whole *modus operandi* of artificial purging; and although, in the latter case, the parts are not adapted to sneezing, yet there is often a dreadful commotion, which has destroyed many thousands of valuable animals. An eminent professor has said that "purgatives, besides being uncertain and uncontrollable, often kill from the dangerous debility they produce." The good results that sometimes appear to follow the exhibition of irritating purges must be attributed to the sanative action of the constitution, and not to the agent itself; and the life of the patient depends, in all cases, on the existing ability of the vital power to counteract the effects of purging, bleeding, poisoning, and blistering.

The author does not wish to give the reader occasion to conclude that purgatives can be entirely dispensed with; on the contrary, he thinks that in many cases they are decidedly beneficial, when given with discretion, and when the nature of the disease requires them; yet even in such cases, too much confidence should not be placed on them, so as to exclude other and sometimes more efficient remedies, which come under the head of laxatives, aperients, &c.

Treatment.—If costiveness is suspected to be symptomatic of some derangement, then a restoration of the general health will establish the lost function of the bowels. In this case, purges are unnecessary; the treatment will altogether depend on the symptoms. For example, suppose the animal constipated; the white of the eye tinged yellow, head drooping, and the animal is drowsy, and off its feed; then give the following:—

Powdered mandrake, ...	1 tea-spoonful.
Castile soap, in shavings, . . .	quarter of an ounce
Beef's gall, ...	half a wine-glass.
Powdered capsicum, ...	third of a table-spoon.

Dissolve the soap in a small quantity of hot water, then mix the whole in three pints of thin gruel.

This makes a good aperient, and can be given with perfect safety in all cases of constipation arising from derangement of the liver. The liquid must be poured down the throat in a gradual manner, in order to insure its reaching the fourth stomach. Aid the medicine by injections, and rub the belly occasionally with straw.

Suppose the bowels to be torpid during an attack of inflammation of the brain; then it will be prudent to combine relaxents and anti-spasmodics, in the following form:—

Extract of butternut, ...	half an ounce.
Powdered skunk cabbage, . . .	"
Cream of tartar, ...	"
Powdered lobelia, ...	2 drachms.

First dissolve the butternut in two quarts of hot water, after which add the remaining ingredients, and give it for a dose. The operation of this prescription, like the preceding, must be aided by injection, friction, and warm drinks made of hyssop or pine boughs.

Suppose the bowels to be constipated, at the same time the animal is hide-bound, in poor condition, &c.; the aperient must then be combined with tonics, as follows:—

Extract of butternut, ...	half an ounce.
Rochelle salts, ...	4 ounces.
Golden seal, ...	1 ounce.
Ginger, ...	1 tea-spoonful.
Hot water, ...	3 quarts.

Dissolve and administer at a dose. In order to relieve the cold, constricted, inactive state of the hide, recourse must be had to warmth, moisture, and friction. A simple aperient of linseed oil may be given in cases of stricture or intussusception of the bowels. The dose is one pint.

FALLING DOWN OF THE FUNDAMENT.

Return the prolapsed part as quickly as possible by gently kneading the parts within the rectum. In recent cases, the part should be washed with an infusion of bayberry bark. (See **Appendix**.) The bowel may be kept in position by applying a wad of cotton, kept wet with the astringent infusion, confined with a bandage. A weak solution of alum water may, however, be substituted, provided the bayberry or white oak bark is not at hand.

Should the parts appear swollen and much inflamed, apply a large slippery elm poultice, on the surface of which sprinkle powdered white oak or bayberry bark. This will soon lessen the swelling, so that the rectum may be returned.

The diet must be very sparing, consisting of flour gruel; and if the bowels are in a relaxed state, add a small quantity of powdered bayberry.

CALVING.

At the end of nine months, the period of the cow's gestation is complete; but parturition does not always take place at that time; it is sometimes earlier, at others later. "One hundred and sixteen cows had their time of calving registered: fourteen of them calved from the two hundred and forty-first day to the two hundred and sixty-sixth day, — that is, eight months and one day to eight months and twenty-six days; fifty-six from the two hundred and seventieth to the two hundred and eightieth day; eighteen from the two hundred and eightieth to the two hundred and ninetieth; twenty on the three hundredth day; five on the three hundred and eighth day; consequently there were sixty-seven days between the two extremities."

Immediately before calving, the animal appears uneasy; the tail is elevated; she shifts from place to place, and is frequently lying down and getting up again. The labor pains then come on; and by the expulsive power of the womb, the fœtus, with the membranes enveloping it, is pushed forward. At first, the membranes appear beyond the vagina, or "shape," often in the form of a bladder of water; the membranes burst, the water is discharged, and the head and fore feet of the calf protrude beyond the shape. We are now supposing a case of natural labor. The body next appears, and soon the delivery is complete. In a short time, a gradual contraction of the womb takes place, and the cleansings (afterbirth) are discharged. When the membranes are ruptured in the early stage of calving, and before the outlet be sufficiently expanded, the process is generally tedious and attended with danger; and this danger arises in part from the premature escape of the fluids contained within the membranes, which are intended, ultimately, to serve the double purpose of expanding or dilating the passage, and lubricating the parts, thereby facilitating the birth.

Under these circumstances, it will be our duty to supply the latter deficiency by carefully anointing the parts with olive oil; at the same time, allow the animal a generous supply of slippery elm gruel: if she refuses to partake of it, when offered in a bucket, it must be gently poured down the throat from a bottle. At times, delivery is very slow; a considerable time elapses before any part of the calf makes its appearance. Here we have only to exercise patience; for if there is a natural presentation, nature, being the best doctor under all circumstances, will do the work in a more faithful manner unassisted than when improperly assisted. "A meddlesome midwifery is bad." Therefore the practice of attempting to hurry the process by driving the animal about, or annoying her in any way, is very improper. In some cases, however, when a wrong presentation is apparent, which seems to render calving impracticable, we should, after smearing the hand with lard, introduce it into the vagina, and endeavor to ascertain the position of the calf, and change it when it is found unfavorable. When, for example, the head presents without the fore legs, which are bent under the breast, we may gently pass the hand along the neck, and, having ascertained the position of the feet, we grasp them, and endeavor to bring them forward, the cow at the same time being put into the most favorable position, viz., the hind quarters being elevated. By this means the calf can be gently pushed back, as the feet are advanced and brought into the outlet. The calf being now in a natural position, we wait patiently, and give nature an opportunity to perform her work. Should the expulsive efforts cease, and the animal appear to be rapidly sinking, no time must be lost; nature evidently calls for assistance, but not in the manner usually resorted to, viz., that of placing a rope around the head and feet of the calf, and employing the united strength of several men to extract the fœtus, without regard to position. Our efforts must be directed to the mother; the calf is a secondary consideration: the strength of the former, if it is failing, must be supported; the expulsive power of the womb and abdominal muscles, now feeble, must be aroused; and there are no means or processes that are better calculated to fulfil these indications than that of administering the following drink: —

Bethroot, ...	2 ounces.
Powdered cayenne, ...	one third of a tea-spoon.
Motherwort, ...	1 ounce.

Infuse in a gallon of boiling water. When cool, strain, then add a gill of honey, and give it in pint doses, as occasion may require.

Under this treatment, there is no difficulty in reëstablishing uterine action. If, however, the labor is still tedious, the calf may be grasped with both hands, and as soon as a pain or expulsive effort is evident, draw the calf from side to side. While making this lateral motion, draw the calf forward. Expulsion generally follows.

If, on examination, it is clearly ascertained that the calf is lying in an unnatural position,—for example, the calf may be in such a position as to present its side across the outlet, —in such cases delivery is not practicable unless the position is altered. Mr. White says, "I have seen a heifer that it was found impossible to deliver. On examining her after death, a very large calf was found lying quite across the mouth of the uterus." In such cases, Mr. Lawson recommends that, "when every other plan has failed for turning the calf, so as to put it in a favorable position for delivery, the following has often succeeded: Let the cow be thrown down in a proper position, and placed on her back; then, by means of ropes and a pulley attached to a beam above, let the hind parts be raised up, so as to be considerably higher than the fore parts; in this position, the calf may be easily put back towards the bottom of the uterus, so as to admit of being turned, or his head and fore legs brought forward without difficulty."

We must ever bear in mind the important fact that the successful termination of the labor depends on the strength and ability of the parent; that if these fail, however successful we may be in bringing about a right presentation, the birth is still tedious, and we may finally have to take the fœtus away piecemeal; by which process the cow's life is put in jeopardy.

To avoid such an unfortunate occurrence, support the animal's strength with camomile tea. The properties of camomile are antispasmodic, carminative, and tonic—just what is wanted.

Mr. White informs us that "instances sometimes occur of the calf's head appearing only, and so large that it is found impossible to put it back. When this is found to be the case, the calf should be killed, and carefully extracted, by cutting off the head and other parts that prevent the extraction; thus the cow's life will be saved."

In cases of malformation of the head of the fœtus, or when the cranium is enormously distended by an accumulation of fluid within the ventricles of the brain, after all other remedies, in the form of fomentations, lubricating antispasmodic drinks, have failed, then recourse must be had to embryotomy.

EMBRYOTOMY.

For the following method of performing the operation we are indebted to Mr. Youatt's work. The details appeared in the London Veterinarian of 1831, and will illustrate the operation. M. Thibeaudeau, the operating surgeon, says, "I was consulted respecting a Breton cow twenty years old, which was unable to calve. I soon discovered the obstacle to the delivery. The fore limbs presented themselves as usual; but the head and neck were turned backwards, and fixed on the left side of the chest, while the fœtus lay on its right side, on the inferior portion of the uterus." M. Thibeaudeau then relates the ineffectual efforts he made to bring the fœtus into a favorable position, and he at length found that his only resource to save the mother was, to cut in pieces the calf, which was now dead. "I amputated the left shoulder of the fœtus," says he, "in spite of the difficulties which the position of the head and neck presented. Having withdrawn the limb, I made an incision through all the cartilages of the ribs, and laid open the chest through its whole extent, by which means I was enabled to extract all the thoracic viscera. Thus having lessened the size of the calf, I was enabled, by pulling at the remaining fore leg, to extract the fœtus without much resistance, although the head and neck were still bent upon the chest. The afterbirth was removed immediately afterwards." This shows the importance of making an early examination, to determine the precise position of the fœtus; for if the head had been discovered in such position in the early stage of labor, it might have been brought forward, and thus prevented the butchery.

FALLING OF THE CALF-BED, OR WOMB.

When much force is used in extracting the calf, it sometimes happens that the womb falls out, or is inverted; and great care is required in putting it back, so that it may remain in that situation.

Treatment.—If the cow has calved during the night, in a cold situation, and, from the exhausted state of the animal, we have reason to suppose that the labor has been tedious, or that she has taken cold, efforts must be made to restore the equilibrium. The following restorative must be given:—

Motherwort tea, ...	2 quarts.
Hot drops, ...	1 table-spoonful.
Powdered cinnamon, ...	1 tea-spoonful.

Give a pint every ten minutes, and support the animal with flour gruel.

The uterus should be returned in the following manner: Place the cow in such a position that the hind parts shall be higher than the fore. Wash the uterus with warm water, into which sprinkle a small quantity of powdered bayberry; remove any extraneous substance from the parts. A linen cloth is then to be put under the womb, which is to be held by two assistants. The cow should be made to rise, if lying down,—that being the most favorable position,—and the operator is then to grasp the mouth of the womb with both hands and return it. When so returned, one hand is to be immediately withdrawn, while the other remains to prevent that part from falling down again. The hand at liberty is then to grasp another portion of the womb, which is to be pushed into the body, like the former, and retained with one hand. This is to be repeated until the whole of the womb is put back. If the womb does not contract, friction, with a brush, around the belly and back, may excite contraction

An attendant must, at the same time, apply a pad wetted with weak alum water to the "shape," and keep it in close contact with the parts, while the friction is going on. It is sometimes necessary to confine the pad by a bandage.

GARGET.

In order to prevent this malady, the calf should be put to suck immediately after the cow has cleansed it; and, if the bag is distended with an overplus of milk, some of it should be milked off. If, however, the teats or quarters become hot and tender, foment with an infusion of elder or camomile flowers, which must be perseveringly applied, at the same time drawing, in the most gentle manner, a small quantity of milk; by which means the over-distended vessels will collapse to their healthy diameter. An aperient must then be given, (see Appendix,) and the animal be kept on a light diet. If there is danger of matter forming, rub the bag with the following liniment: —

Goose oil, ... } equal parts.
Hot drops, ... }

If the parts are exceedingly painful, wash with a weak lie, or wood ashes, or sal soda. In spite of all our efforts, matter will sometimes form. As soon as it is discovered, a lancet may be introduced, and the matter evacuated; then wash the part clean, and apply the stimulating liniment. (See Appendix)

SORE TEATS.

First wash with castile soap and warm water; then apply the following: —

Lime water,	. . . .	equal parts.
Linseed oil,	. . . .	

CHAPPED TEATS AND CHAFED UDDER.

These may be treated in the same manner.

If the above preparation is not at hand, substitute bayberry tallow, elder or marshmallow ointment.

FEVER.

Description and Definition. — Fever is a powerful effort of the vital principle to expel from the system morbific or irritating matter, or to bring about a healthy action. The reason why veterinary practitioners have not ascertained this fact heretofore is, because they have been guided by false principles, to the exclusion of their own common experience. Let them receive the truth of the definition we have given; then the light will begin to shine, and medical darkness will be rendered more visible. Fever, we have said, is a vital action — an effort of the vital power to regain its equilibrium of action through the system, and should never be subdued by the use of the lancet, or any destructive agents that deprive the organs of the power to produce it. Fever will be generally manifested in one or more of that combination of signs known as follows: loss of appetite, increased velocity of the pulse, difficult respiration, heaving at the flank, thirst, pain, and swelling; some of which will be present, local or general in greater or less degree, in all forms of disease. When an animal has taken cold, and there is power in the system to keep up a continual warfare against encroachments, the disturbance of vital action being unbroken, the fever is called pure or persistent. Emanations from animal or vegetable substances in a state of decomposition or putrefaction, or the noxious miasmata from marshy lands, if concentrated, and not sufficiently diluted with atmospheric air, enter into the system, and produce a specific effect. In order to dethrone the intruder, who keeps up a system of aggression from one tissue to another, the vital power arrays her artillery, in good earnest, to resist the invading foe ; and if furnished with the munitions of war in the form of sanative agents, she generally conquers the enemy, and dictates her own terms. While the forces are equally balanced, which may be known by a high grade of vital action, it is also called *unbroken* or *pure* fever. The powers of the system may become exhausted by efforts at relief, and the fever will be periodically reduced; this form of fever is called *remittent*. By remittent fever is to be understood this modification of vital action which rests or abates, but does not go entirely off before a fresh attack ensues. It is evident, in this case, also, that nature is busily engaged in the work of establishing her empire ; but being more exhausted, she occasionally rests from her labors. It would be as absurd to expect that the most accurate definition of fever in one animal would correspond in all its details with another case, as to expect all animals to be alike. There are many names given to fevers ; for example, in addition to the two already alluded to, we have milk or puerperal fever, symptomatic, typhus, inflammatory, &c. Veterinary Surgeon Percival, in an article on fever, says, "We have no more reason — not near so much — to give fever a habitation in the abdomen, than we have to enthrone it in the head ; but it would appear from the full range of observation, that no part of the body can be said to be unsusceptible of inflammation, (local fever,) though, at the same time, no organ is invariably or exclusively affected."

From this we learn that disease always attacks the weak

est organ, and that our remedies should be adapted to act on all parts of the system.

The same author continues, "All I wish to contend for is, that both idiopathic and symptomatic fevers exhibit the same form, character, species, and the same general means of cure; and that, were it not for the local affection, it would be difficult or impossible to distinguish them."

Fever has always been the great bugbear, to scare the farmer and cattle doctor into a wholesale system of blood-letting and purging; they believe that the more fever the animal manifests, the more unwearied must be their exertions. The author advises the farmer not to feel alarmed about the fever; for when that is present it shows that the vital principle is up and doing. Efforts should be made to open the outlets of the body, through which the morbific materials may pass: the fever will then subside. It will be difficult to make the community credit this simple truth, because fever is quite a fashionable disease, and it is an easy matter to make the farmer believe that his cow has a very peculiar form of it, that requires an entirely different mode of treatment from that of another form. Then it is very profitable to the interested allopathic doctor, who can produce any amount of "learned nonsense" to justify the ways and means, and support his theory.

The author does not wish, at the present time, to enter into a learned discussion of the merit or demerit of allopathy: the object of this work is, to impart practical information to farmers and owners of stock. In order to accomplish this object, an occasional reference to the absurdities of the old school is unavoidable.

A celebrated writer has said, "The very medicines [meaning those used by the old school, which kill more than they ever cure] which aggravate and protract the malady bind a laurel on the doctor's brow. When, at last, the sick are saved by the living powers of nature struggling against death and the physician, he receives all the credit of a miraculous cure; he is lauded to the skies for delivering the sick from the details of the most deadly symptoms of misery into which he himself had plunged them, and out of which they never would have arisen, but by the restorative efforts of that living power which at once triumphed over poison, blood-letting, disease, and death."

In the treatment of disease, and when fever is manifested by the signs just enumerated, the object is, to invite the blood to the external surface; or, in other words, equalize the circulation by warmth and moisture; give diaphoretic or sudorific medicines, (see APPENDIX,) with a view of relaxing the capillary structure, ridding the system of morbific materials, and allaying the general excitement. If the ears and legs are cold, rub them diligently with a brush; if they again relapse into a cold state, rub them with stimulating liniment and bandage them with flannel. In short, to contract, to stimulate, remove obstructions, and furnish the system with the materials for self-defence, are the means to be resorted to in the cure of fevers.

We shall now give a few examples of the treatment of fever; from which the reader will form some idea of the course to be pursued in other forms not enumerated. But we may be asked why we make so many divisions of fever when it is evidently a unit. We answer the question in the words of Professor Curtis, whose teachings first emancipated us from the absurdity of allopathic theories. "These divisions were made by the learned in physic, and we follow them out in their efforts to divide what is in its nature indivisible, to satisfy the demands of the public, and to give it in small crums to those practitioners of the art who have not capacity enough to take in the whole at a single mouthful."

In the treatment of fevers, we must endeavor to remove all intruding agents, their influences and effects, and reëstablish a full, free, and universal equilibrium throughout the system. "The means are," says Professor Curtis, "antispasmodics, stimulants, and tonics, with emollients to grease the wheels of life. Disprove these positions, and we lay by the pen and 'throw physic to the dogs.' Adhere strictly to them in the use of the best means, and you will do all that can be done in the hour of need."

MILK OR PUERPERAL FEVER.

Treatment. — Aperients are exceedingly important in the early stages, for they liberate any offending matter that may have accumulated in the different compartments of the stomach or intestines, and deplete the system with more certainty and less danger than blood-letting.

Aperient for Puerperal Fever.

Rochelle salts, ...	4 ounces.
Manna, ...	2 ounces.
Extract of butternut, ...	half an ounce.
Dissolve in boiling water, . . .	3 quarts.

To be given at a dose.

By the aid of one or more of the following drinks, the aperient will generally operate: —

Give a bountiful supply of hyssop tea, sweetened with honey. Keep the surface warm.

Suppose the secretion of milk to be arrested; then apply warm fomentations to the udder.

Suppose the bowels to be torpid; then use injections of soap-suds and salt.

Suppose the animal to be in poor condition; then give the following: —

Powdered balmony or gentian, . .	1 ounce.
Golden seal, ...	1 ounce.
Flour gruel, ...	1 gallon.

To be given in quart doses, every four hours.

Suppose the bowels to be distended with gas; then give the following: —

Powdered caraways, ...	1 ounce.
Assafœtida, ...	1 tea-spoonful.
Boiling water, ...	2 quarts.

To be given at a dose.

Any of the above preparations may be repeated, as circumstances seem to require. Yet it must be borne in mind that we are apt to do too much, and that the province of the good physician is "to know when to do nothing." The following case from Mr. Youatt's work illustrates this fact: —

"A very singular variety of milk fever has already been hinted at. The cow is down, but there is apparently nothing more the matter with her than that she is unable to rise; she eats and drinks, and ruminates as usual, and the evacuations are scarcely altered. In this state she continues from ten days to a fortnight, and then she gets up well." Yes, and many thousands more would "get up well," if they were only let alone. Nature requires assistance sometimes: hence the need of doctors and nurses. All, however, that is required of the doctor to do is, just to attend to the calls of nature, — whose servant he is, — and bring her what she wants to use in her own way. The nearer the remedies partake or consist of air, water, warmth, and food, the more sure and certain are they to do good.

If a cow, in high condition, has just calved, appears restless, becomes irritable, the eye and tongue protruding, and a total suspension of milk takes place, we may conclude that there is danger of puerperal fever. No time should be lost: the aperient must be given immediately; warm injections must be thrown into the rectum, and the teats must be industriously drawn, to solicit the secretion of milk. In this case, all food should be withheld: "starve a fever" suits this case exactly.

INFLAMMATORY FEVER.

Inflammatory fever manifests itself very suddenly. The animal may appear well during the day, but at night it appears dull, refuses its food, heaves at the flanks, seems uneasy, and sometimes delirious; the pulse is full and bounding; the mouth hot; urine high colored and scanty. Sometimes there are hot and cold stages.

Remarks. — When disease attacks any particular organ suddenly, or in an acute form, inflammatory fever generally manifests itself. Now, disease may attack the brain, the lungs, kidneys, spleen, bowels, pleura, or peritoneum. Inflammatory fever may be present in each case. Now, it is evident that the fever is not the real enemy to be overcome; it is only a manifestation of disorder, not the cause of it. The skin may be obstructed, thereby retaining excrementitious materials in the system: the reabsorption of the latter produces fever; hence it is obvious that a complete cure can only be effected by the removal of its causes, or, rather, the restoration of the suppressed evacuations, secretions, or excretions.

It is very important that we observe and imitate nature in her method of curing fever, which is, the restoration of the secretions, and, in many cases, by sweat, or by diarrhœa; either of which processes will remove the irritating or offending cause, and promote equilibrium of action throughout the whole animal system. In fulfilling these indications consists the whole art of curing fever.

But says one, "It is a very difficult thing to sweat an ox." Then the remedies should be more perseveringly applied. Warm, relaxing, antispasmodic drinks should be freely allowed, and these should be aided by warmth, moisture, and friction externally; and by injection, if needed. If the ox does not actually sweat under this system of medication, he will throw off a large amount of insensible perspiration.

Causes. — In addition to the causes already enumerated, are the accumulation of excrementitious and morbific materials in the system. Dr. Eberle says, "A large proportion of the recrementitious elements of perspirable matter must, when the surface is obstructed, remain and mingle with the blood, (unless speedily removed by the vicarious action of some other emunctory,) and necessarily impart to this fluid qualities that are not natural to it. Most assuredly the retention of materials which have become useless to the system, and for whose constant elimination nature has provided so extensive a series of emunctories as the cutaneous exhalents, cannot be long tolerated by the animal economy with entire impunity."

Dr. White says, "Many of the diseases of horses and cattle are caused by suppressed or checked perspiration; the various appearances they assume depending, perhaps, in a great measure, upon the suddenness with which this discharge is stopped, and the state of the animal at the time it takes place.

"Cattle often suffer from being kept in cold, bleak situations, particularly in the early part of spring, during the prevalence of an easterly wind; in this case, the suppression of the discharge is more gradual, and the diseases which result from it are slower in their progress, consequently more insidious in their nature; and it often happens that the animal is left in the same cold situation until the disease is incurable."

It seems probable that, in these cases, the perspiratory vessels gradually lose their power, and that, at length, a total and permanent suppression of that necessary discharge takes place; hence arise inflammatory fever, consumption, decayed liver, rot, mesenteric obstructions, and various other complaints. How necessary, therefore, is it for proprietors of cattle to be provided with sheltered situations for their stock! How many diseases might they prevent by such precaution, and how much might they save, not only in preserving the lives of their cattle, but in avoiding the expense (too often useless, to say the least of it) of cattle doctoring!

Treatment. — We first give an aperient, (see APPENDIX,) to deplete the system. The common practice is to deplete by blood-letting, which only protracts the malady, and often brings on typhus, black quarter, joint murrain, &c. Promote the secretions and excretions in the manner already referred to under the head of *Puerperal Fever;* this will relieve the stricture of the surface. A drink made from either of the following articles should be freely given: lemon balm, wardering milk weed, thoroughwort, or lady's slipper, made as follows: —

Take either of the above articles, . . .	2 ounces.
Boiling water, ...	2 quarts.

When cool, strain, and add a wine-glass of honey.

If there is great thirst, and the mouth is hot and dry, the animal may have a plentiful supply of water.

If the malady threatens to assume a putrid or malignant type, add a small quantity of capsicum and charcoal to the drink, and support the strength of the animal with flour gruel.

TYPHUS FEVER

Causes. — Sudden changes in the temperature of the atmosphere, the animal being at the same time in a state of debility, unable to resist external agencies.

Treatment. — Support the powers of the system through the means of nutritious diet, in the form of flour gruel, scalded meal and shorts, bran-water, &c.

Give tonics, relaxents, and antispasmodics, in the following form: —

Powdered capsicum, ...	1 tea-spoonful.
" bloodroot, ...	1 ounce.
" cinnamon, ...	half an ounce.
Thoroughwort or valerian, . . .	2 ounces.
Boiling water, ...	1 gallon.

When cold, strain, and give a quart every two hours.

Remove the contents of the rectum by injections of a stimulating character, and invite action to the extremities by rubbing them with stimulating liniment, (which see.) A drink of camomile tea should be freely allowed; if diarrhœa sets in, add half a tea-spoon of bayberry bark to every two quarts of the tea.

These few examples of the treatment of fever will give

the farmer an idea of the author's manner of treating it, who can generally break up a fever in a few hours, whereas the popular method of "smothering the fire," as Mr. Youatt terms the blood-letting process, instead of curing, will produce all forms of fever. Here is a specimen of the treatment, in fever of a putrid type, recommended by Dr. Brocklesby. He says, "Immediately upon refusing fodder, the beast should have three quarts of blood taken away; and after twelve hours, two quarts more; after the next twelve hours, about three pints may be let out; and after the following twelve hours, diminish a pint of blood from the quantity taken away at the preceding blood-letting; lastly, about a single pint should be taken away in less than twelve hours after the former bleeding; so that, when the beast has been blooded five times, in the manner here proposed, the worst symptoms will, it is hoped, abate; but if the difficulty and panting for breath continue very great, I see no reason against repeated bleeding." (See Lawson's work on cattle, p. 312.) The author has consulted several authorities on the treatment of typhus, and finds that the use of the lancet is invariably recommended. We do not expect to find, among our American farmers, any one so reckless, so lost to the common feelings of humanity, and his own interest, as to follow out the directions here given by Dr. B.; still blood-letting is practised, to some extent, in every section of the Union, and will continue to be the sheet-anchor of the cattle doctor just so long as the influential and cattle-rearing community shall be kept in darkness as to its destructive tendency. Unfortunately for the poor dumb brute, veterinary writers have from time immemorial been uncompromising advocates for bleeding; and through the influence which their talents and position confer, they have wielded the medical sceptre with a despotism worthy of a better cause. It were a bootless task to attempt to reform the disciples of allopathy; for, if you deprive them of the lancet, and their *materia medica* of poisons, they cannot practise. They must be reformed through public opinion; and for this purpose we publish our own experience, and that of others who have dared to assail allopathy, with the mora certainty that they would expose themselves to contempt, and be branded as "medical heretics."

No treatment is scientific, in the estimation of some, unless it includes the lancet, firing-iron, setons, boring horns, cramming down salts by the pound, and castor oil by the quart. The object of this work is to correct this erroneous notion, and show the *farming community* that a safer and more efficient system of medication has just sprung into existence. When the principles of this reformed system of medication are understood and practised, then the veterinary science will be a very different thing from what it has heretofore been, and men will hail it as a blessing instead of a "curse." They will then know the power that really cures, and devise means of prevention. And here, reader, permit us to introduce the opinions of an able advocate of reform in human practice:* the same remarks apply to cattle; for they are governed by the same universal laws that we are, and whether we prescribe for a man or an ox, the laws of the animal economy are the same, and require that the same indications shall be fulfilled.

"A little examination into the consequences of blood-letting will prove that, so far from its being beneficial, it is productive of the most serious effects.

"Nature has endowed the animal frame with the power of preparing, from proper aliment, a certain quantity of blood. This vital fluid, subservient to nutrition, is, by the amazing structure of the heart and blood-vessels, circulated through the different parts of the system. A certain natural balance between what is taken in and what passes off by the several outlets of the body is, in a state of health, regularly preserved. When this balance, so essential to health and life, is, contrary to the laws of the animal constitution, interrupted, either a deviation from a sound state is immediately perceived, or health from that moment is rendered precarious

* Dr. Beach.

Blood-letting tends artificially to destroy the natural balance in the constitution." (For more important information on blood-letting, see the author's work on the Horse; also page 58 of the present volume.)

HORN AIL IN CATTLE.

On applying the hand to the horn or horns of a sick beast, an unnatural heat, or sometimes coldness, is felt: this enables us to judge of the degree of sympathetic disturbance. And here, reader, permit us to protest against a cruel practice, that is much in fashion, viz., that of boring the horns with a gimlet; for it does not mend the matter one jot, and at best it is only treating symptoms. The gimlet frequently penetrates the frontal sinuses which communicate with the nasal passages, and where mucous secretion, if vitiated or tenacious, will accumulate. On withdrawing the gimlet, a small quantity of thick mucus, often blood, escapes, and the interested operator will probably bore the other horn. Now, it often happens that after the point of the gimlet has passed through one side of the horn and bony structure, it suddenly enters a sinus, and does not meet with any resistance until it reaches the opposite side. Many a "mare's nest" has been found in this way, usually announced as follows: "The horn is hollow!" Again, in aged animals, the bony structure within the horn often collapses or shrinks, forming a sinus or cavity within the horn: by boring in a lateral direction, the gimlet enters it; the horn is then pronounced hollow! and, according to the usual custom, must be doctored. An abscess will sometimes form in the frontal sinuses, resulting from common catarrh or "hoose;" the gimlet may penetrate the sac containing the pus, which thus escapes; but it would escape, finally, through the nostrils, if it were let alone. Here, again, the "horns are diseased;" and should the animal recover, (which it would, eventually, without any interference,) the recovery is strangely attributed to the boring process. An author, whose name has escaped our memory, recommends "cow doctors to carry a gimlet in their pocket." We say to such men, Lead yourselves not into temptation! if you put a gimlet into your pocket, you will be very likely to slip it into the cow's horn. Some men have a kind of instinctive impulse to bore the cow's horns; we allude to those who are unacquainted with the fact that "horn ail" is only a symptom of derangement. It is no more a disease of the horns than it is of the functions generally; for if there be an excess or deficiency of vital action within or around the base of the horn, there must be a corresponding deficiency or excess, as the case may be, in some other region.

"Horn ail," as it is improperly termed, we have said, may accompany common catarrh, also that of an epidemic form; the horns will feel unnatural if there be a determination of blood to the head: this might be easily equalized by stimulating the external surface and extremities, at the same time giving antispasmodic teas and regulating the diet. The horns will feel cold whenever there is an unnatural distribution of the blood, and this may arise from exposure, or suffering the animal to wallow in filth. The author has been consulted in many cases of "horn ail," in several of which there were slow fecal movements, or constipation; the conjunctiva of the eyes were injected with yellow fluid, and of course a deficiency of bile in the abomasum, or fourth stomach; thus plainly showing that the animals were laboring under derangement of the digestive organs. Our advice was, to endeavor to promote a healthy action through the whole system; to stimulate the digestive organs; to remove obstructions, both by injection, if necessary, and by the use of aperients; lastly, to invite action to the extremities, by stimulating liniments Whenever these indications are fulfilled, "horn ail" soon disappears.

ABORTION IN COWS.

Cows are particularly liable to the accident of "slinking the calf." The common causes of abortion are, the respiration and ultimate absorption of emanations from putrid animal remains, miasmata, over-feeding, derangement of the stomach, &c. The filthy, stagnant water they are often compelled to drink is likewise a serious cause, not only of abortion, but also of general derangement of the animal functions. Dr. White, V. S., tells us that "a farm in England had been given up three successive times in consequence of the loss the owners sustained by abortion in their cattle. At length the fourth proprietor, after suffering considerably in losses occasioned by abortion in his stock, suspected that the water of his ponds, which was extremely filthy, might be the cause of the mischief. He therefore dug three wells upon his farm, and, having fenced round the pond to prevent the cattle from drinking there, caused them to be supplied with the well water, in stone troughs erected for the purpose; and from this moment the evil was remedied, and the quality of the butter and cheese made on his farm was greatly improved. In order to show," says the same author, "that the accident of abortion may arise from a vitiated state of the digestive organs, I will here notice a few circumstances tending to corroborate this opinion. In 1782, all the cows of the farmer D'Euruse, in Picardy, miscarried. The period at which they warped was about the fourth or fifth month. The accident was attributed to the excessive heat of the preceding summer; but, as the water they were in the habit of drinking was extremely bad, and they had been kept on oat, wheat, and rye straw, it appears to me more probable, that the great quantity of straw they were obliged to eat, in order to obtain sufficient nourishment, and the injury sustained by the third stomach in expressing the fluid parts of the masticated or ruminated mass, together with the large quantity of water they drank, while kept on this dry food, were the real causes of the miscarriage.

"A farmer at Chariton, out of a dairy of twenty-eight cows, had sixteen slip their calves at different periods of gestation The summer had been very dry; they had been pastured in muddy place, which was flooded by the Seine. Here the cows were generally up to their knees in mud and water. In 1789, all the cows in a village near Mantes miscarried. All the lands in this place were so stiff as to be, for some time, impervious to water; and as a vast quantity of rain fell that year, the pastures were for a time completely inundated, on which account the grass became bad. This proves that keeping cows on food that is deficient in nutritive properties, and difficult of digestion, is one of the principal causes of miscarriage." Mr. Youatt says, "It is supposed that the sight of a slipped calf, or the smell of putrid animal substances, are apt to produce warping. Some curious cases of abortion, which are worthy of notice, happened in the dairy of a French farmer. For thirty years his cows had been subject to abortion. His cow-house was large and well ventilated; his cows were in apparent health; they were fed like others in the village; they drank the same water; there was nothing different in the pasture; he had changed his servants many times in the course of thirty years; he pulled down the barn and cow-house, and built another, on a different plan; he even, agreeably to superstition, took away the aborted calf through the window, that the curse of future abortion might not be entailed on the cow that passed over the same threshold. To make all sure, he had broken through the wall at the end of the cow-house, and opened a new door. But still the trouble continued. Several of his cows had died in the act of abortion, and he had replaced them by others; many had been sold, and their vacancies filled up. He was advised to make a thorough change. This had never occurred to him; but at once he saw the propriety of the counsel. He sold every beast, and the pest was stayed, and never appeared in his new stock. This was owing, probably, to sympathetic influence:

the result of such influence is as fatal as the direst contagion."

My own opinion of this disease is, that it is one of nervous origin; that there is a loss of equilibrium between the nerves of voluntary and involuntary motion. The direct causes of this pathological state exist in any thing that can derange the organs of digestion. Great sympathy is known to exist between the organs of generation and the stomach: if the latter be deranged, the former feels a corresponding influence, and the sympathetic nerves are the media by which the change takes place.

It invariably follows that, as soon as impregnation takes place, the stomach from that moment takes on an irritable state, and is more susceptible to the action of unfavorable agents. Thus the odor of putrid substances causes nausea or relaxation when the animal is in a state of pregnancy; otherwise, the same odor would not affect it in the least. Professor Curtis says, "The nervous system constitutes the check lines by which the vital spirit governs, as a coachman does his horses, the whole motive apparatus of the animal economy; that every line, or pencil, or ganglion of lines, in it, is antagonistic to some other line or ganglion, so that, whenever the function of one is exalted, that of some other is depressed. It follows, of course, that to equalize the nervous action, and to sustain the equilibrium, is one of the most important duties of the physician."

In addition to the causes of abortion already enumerated, we may add violent exercise, jumping dikes or hedges, sudden frights, and blows or bruises.

Treatment. — When a cow has slipped her fœtus, and appears in good condition, the quantity of food usually given should be lessened. Give the following drink every night for a week: —

Valerian, (herb,)	1 ounce.
Powdered skunk cabbage, . .	1 tea-spoonful.

Steep in half a gallon of boiling water. When cold, strain and administer.

Suppose the animal to be in poor condition; then put her on a nourishing diet, and give tonics and stimulants, as follows:—

Powdered gentian, ...	1 ounce.
" sassafras, ...	1 ounce.
Linseed or flaxseed, ...	1 pound.

Mix. Divide into six portions, and give one, night and morning, in the food, which ought to consist of scalded meal and shorts. A sufficient quantity of hay should be allowed; yet grass will be preferable, if the season permits.

Suppose the animal to have received an injury; then rest and a scalded diet are all that are necessary. As a means of prevention, see article *Feeding*, page 17.

COW-POX.

This malady makes its appearance on the cow's teats in the form of small pustules, which, after the inflammatory stage, suppurate. A small quantity of matter then escapes, and forms a crust over the circumference of each pustule. If the crust be suffered to remain until new skin is formed beneath, they will heal without any interference. It often happens, however, that, in the process of milking, the scabs are rubbed off. The following wash must then be resorted to:—

Pyroligneous acid, ...	a wine-glass.
Water, ...	1 pint.

Wet the parts two or three times a day; medicine is unnecessary. A few meals of scalded food will complete the cure

---

MANGE.

"Mange may be generated either from excitement of the skin itself, or through the medium of that sympathetic influence which is known to exist between the skin and organs of digestion. We have, it appears to me, an excellent illustration of this in the case of mange supervening upon poverty — a fact too notorious to be disputed, though there may be different ways of theorizing on it."

Mr. Blanie says, "Mange has three origins — filth, debility, and contagion."

Treatment. — Rid the system of morbific materials with the following: —

Powdered sassafras, ...	2 ounces.
" charcoal, ...	a handful.
Sulphur, ...	1 ounce.

Mix, and divide into six parts; one to be given in the feed, night and morning. The daily use of the following wash will then complete the cure, provided proper attention be paid to the diet.

Wash for Mange.

Pyroligneous acid, ...	4 ounces.
Water, ...	a pint.

The mange is known to be infectious: this suggests the propriety of removing the animal from the rest of the herd.

HIDE-BOUND

THIS is seldom, if ever, a primary disease The known sympathy existing between the digestive organs and the skin enables us to trace the malady to acute or chronic indigestion.

Treatment. — The indications to be fulfilled are, to invite action to the surface by the aid of warmth, moisture, friction, and stimulants, to tone up the digestive organs, and relax the whole animal. The latter indications are fulfilled by the use of the following: —

Powdered balmony, (snakehead,) . .	2 ounces.
" sassafras, ...	1 ounce.
Linseed, ...	2 pounds.
Sulphur, ...	1 ounce.

Mix together, and divide the mass into eight equal parts, and give one night and morning, in scalded shorts or meal; the better way, however, is, to turn it down the throat.

A few boiled carrots should be allowed, especially in the winter season, for they possess peculiar remedial properties, which are generally favorable to the cure.

LICE.

Treatment. — Wash the skin, night and morning, with the following: —

Powdered lobelia seeds.	2 ounces.
Boiling water, ...	1 quart.

After standing a few hours, it is fit for use, and can be applied with a sponge.

IMPORTANCE OF KEEPING THE SKIN OF ANIMALS IN A HEALTHY STATE.

This is a subject of great importance to the farmer: for many of the diseases of cattle arise from the filthy, obstructed state of the surface. This neglect of cleansing the hide of cattle arises, in some cases, from the absurd notion (often expressed to the author) that the hide of cattle is so thick and dense that they never sweat, except on the muzzle! For the information of those who may have formed such an absurd and dangerous notion, we give the views of Professor Bouley. "In all animals, from the exterior tegumentary surface incessantly exhale vaporous or gaseous matters, the products of chemical operations going on in the interior of the organism, of which the uninterrupted elimination is a necessary condition for the regular continuance of the functions. Regarded in this point of view, the skin may be considered as a dependency of the respiratory apparatus, of which it continues and completes the function, by returning incessantly to the atmosphere the combusted products, which are water and carbonic acid.

"Therefore the skin, properly speaking, is an expiratory apparatus, which, under ordinary conditions of the organism, exhales, in an insensible manner, products analogous to those expired from the pulmonary surface; with this difference, that the quantity of carbonic acid is very much less considerable in the former than in the latter of these exhalations; according to Burbach, the proportion of carbonic acid, as inhaled by the skin, being to that expired by the lungs as 350 to 23,450, or as 1 to 67.

"The experiments made on inferior animals, such as frogs, toads, salamanders, or fish, have demonstrated the waste by general transpiration to be, in twenty-four hours, little less than half the entire weight of the body."

The same author remarks, "Direct experiment has shown,

in the clearest manner, the close relation of function existing between the perspiratory and respiratory membranes."

"M. Fourcault, with a view of observing, through different species of animals, the effect of the suppression of perspiration, conceived the notion of having the skins of certain live animals covered with varnish. After having been suitably prepared, some by being plucked, others by being shorn, he smeared them with varnish of variable composition; the substances employed being tar, paste, glue, pitch, and other plastic matters. Sometimes these, one or more of them, were spread upon parts, sometimes upon the whole of the body. The effects of the operation have varied, showing themselves, soon or late afterwards, decisively or otherwise, according as the varnishing has been complete or general, or only partial, thick, thin, &c. In every instance, the health of the animal has undergone strange alterations, and life has been grievously compromised. Those that have been submitted to experiment under our eyes have succumbed in one, two, three days, and even at the expiration of some hours." (See *London Veterinarian* for 1850, p. 353.)

In a subsequent number of the same work we find the subject resumed; from which able production we select the following: —

"The suppression of perspiration has at all times been thought to have a good deal to do with the production of disease. Without doubt this has been exaggerated. But allowing this exaggeration, is it not admitted by all practitioners that causes which act through the medium of the skin are susceptible, in sufficient degree, of being appreciated in the circumstances ushering in the development of very many diseases, especially those characterized by any active flux of the visceral organs? For example, is it not an incontestable pathological fact, that catarrhal, bronchial, pulmonic, and pleuritic affections, congestions of the most alarming description in the vascular abdominal system of the horse, inflammation of the peritoneum and womb following labor, catarrhal inflammations of the bowels, even congestions of the feet, &c., derive their origin, in a great number of instances, from cold applied to the skin in a state of perspiration? What happens in the organism after the application of such a cause? Is its effect instantaneous? Let us see. Immediately on the repercussive action of cold being felt by the skin, the vascular system of internal parts finds itself filled with repelled blood. Though this effect, however, be simply hydrostatic, the diseased phenomena consecutive on it are far otherwise.

"It is quite certain that, in the immense system of communicating vessels forming the circulating apparatus, whenever any large quantity of blood flows to any one particular part of the body, the other vessels of the system must be comparatively empty.* The knowledge of this organic hydrostatic fact it is that has given origin to the use of revulsives under their various forms, and we all well know how much service we derive from their use.

"But in what does this diseased condition consist? Whereabouts is it seated?

"The general and undefined mode it has of showing its presence in the organism points this out. Immediately subsequent to the action of the cause, the actual seat of the generative condition of the disease about to appear is the blood; this fluid it is which, having become actually modified in its chemical compositions under the influence of the cause that has momentarily obstructed the cutaneous exhalations, carries about every where with it the disordered condition, and ultimately giving rise, through it, to some local disease, as a sort of eruptive effort, analogous in its object, but often less salutary in its effect; owing to the functional importance of the part attacked, to the external eruptions produced by the pres-

* What a destructive system, then, must blood-letting be, which proposes to supply this deficiency in the empty vessels by opening a vein and suffering the contents of the overcharged vessels to fall to the ground! If the blood abstracted from the full veins could be returned into those "empty" ones, then there would be some sense in blood-letting.

ence in the blood of virus, which alters both its dynamic and chemical properties.

"But what is the nature of this alteration? In this case, every clew to the solution of this question fails us. We know well, when the experiment is designedly prolonged, the blood grows black, as in *asphyxia*, (loss of pulse,) through the combination with it of carbonic acid, whose presence is opposed to the absorption of oxygen. But what relation is there between this chemical alteration of blood here and the modifications in composition it may undergo under the influence of instantaneous suppression, but not persistent, of the cutaneous exhalations and secretions? The experiments of Dr. Fourcault tend, on the whole, to explain this. His experiments discover the primitive form and almost the nature of the alteration the blood undergoes under the influence of the cessation of the functions of the skin. They demonstrate that under these conditions the regularity of the course of this fluid is disturbed — that it has a tendency to accumulate and stagnate within the internal organs: witness the abdominal pains so frequently consequent on the application of plasters upon the skin, and the congestions of the abdominal and pulmonary vascular systems met with almost always on opening animals which have been suffocated through tar or pitch plasters.

"They prove, in fact, the thorough aptitude of impression of the nervous system to blood altered in its chemical properties, while they afford us an explication of the phenomena of depression, and muscular prostration, and weakness, which accompany the beginning of disease consecutive on the operation of cold.

"How often do we put a stop to the ulterior development of disease by restoring the function of the skin by mere [dry] friction, putting on thick clothing, exposing to exciting fumigation, applying temporary revulsives in the shape of mustard poultices, administering diffusible stimuli made warm in drenches, trying every means to force the skin, and so tend, by the reëstablishment of its exhalent functions, to permit the elimination of blood saturated with carbonic matters opposed to the absorption by it of oxygen!

"Do we not here perceive, so to express ourselves, the evil enter and depart through the skin?

"M. Roche-Lubin gives an account of some lambs which were exposed, after being shorn, to a humid icy cold succeeding upon summer heat. These animals all died; and their post mortem examination disclosed nothing further than a blackened condition of blood throughout the whole circulating system, with stagnation in some organs, such as the liver the spleen, or abdominal vascular system.

"From the foregoing disclosures, which might be multiplied if there was need of it, we learn that the regularity or perversion of the functions of the skin exercises an all-powerful influence over the conservation or derangement of the health, and that very many diseases can be traced to no other origin than the interruption, more or less, of these functions."

These remarks are valuable, inasmuch as they go to prove the importance, in the treatment of disease, of a restoration of the lost function. Our system of applying friction, warmth, and moisture to the external surface, in all cases of internal disease, here finds, in the authors just quoted, able advocates

SPAYING COWS.

The castration of cows has been practised for several years in different parts of the world, with such remarkable success, that no one will doubt there are advantages to be derived from it. For the benefit of those who may have doubts on this subject, we give the opinions of a committee appointed by the Rheims Academy to investigate the matter.

"To the question put to the committee —

"1st. Is the spaying of cows a dangerous operation?

"The answer is, This operation, in itself, involves no more

danger than many others of as bold a character, (as puncture of the rumen,) which are performed without accident by men even strangers to the veterinary art. Two minutes suffice for the extraction of the ovaries; two minutes more for suturing the wound.

"2dly. Will not the spaying of cows put an end to the production of the species?

"Without doubt, this is an operation which must be kept within bounds. It is in the vicinity of large towns that most benefit will be derived from it, where milk is most generally sought after, and where pasturage is scanty, and consequently food for cows expensive. On this account it is not the practice to raise calves about the environs of Paris. Indeed, at Cormenteul, near Rheims, out of one hundred and forty-five cows kept, not more than from ten to fifteen calves are produced yearly.

"3dly. Is spaying attended with amelioration of the quality of the meat?

"That cows fatten well after being spayed is an incontestable fact, long known to agriculturists.

"4thly. Does spaying prolong the period of lactation, and increase the quantity of milk?

"The cow will be found to give as much milk after eighteen months as immediately after the operation; and there was found in quantity, in favor of the spayed cows, a great difference.

"5thly. Is the quality of the milk ameliorated by spaying?

"To resolve this question, we have thought proper to make an appeal to skilful chemists resident in the neighborhood; and they have determined that the milk abounds more by one third in cheese and butter than that of ordinary cows."

Mr. Percival says, "No person hesitates to admit the advantages derivable from the castration of bulls and stallions. I do not hesitate to aver, that equal, if not double, advantages are to be derived from the same operation when performed on cows."

"It is to America we are indebted for this discovery. In

1832, an American traveller, a lover of milk, no doubt, asked for some of a farmer at whose house he was. Surprised at finding at this farm better milk than he had met with elsewhere, he wished to know the reason of it. After some hesitation, the farmer avowed, that he had been advised to perform on his cows the same operation as was practised on the bulls. The traveller was not long in spreading this information. The Veterinary Society of the country took up the discovery, when it got known in America. The English — those ardent admirers of beefsteaks and roast beef — profited by the new procedure, as they know how to turn every thing to account, and at once castrated their heifers, in order to obtain a more juicy meat.

"The Swiss, whose principal employment is agricultural, had the good fortune to possess a man distinguished in his art, who foresaw, and was anxious to realize, the advantages of castrating milch cows. M. Levrat, veterinary surgeon at Lausanne, found in the government of his country an enlightened assistant in his praiseworthy and useful designs, so that, at the present day, instructions in the operation of spaying enter into the requirements of the programme of the professors of agriculture, and the gelders of the country are not permitted to exercise their calling until they have proved their qualifications on the same point." — *London Vet.* p. 274, 1850.

For additional evidence in favor of spaying, see Albany Cultivator, p. 145, vol. vi.

We have conversed with several farmers in this section of the United States, and find, as a general thing, that they labor under the impression that spaying is chiefly resorted to with a view of fattening cattle for the market. We have, on all occasions, endeavored to correct this erroneous conclusion, and at the same time to point out the benefits to be derived from this practice. The quality of the milk is superior, and the quantity is augmented. Many thousands of the miserable specimens of cows, that the farmer, with all his care, and having, at the same time an abundance of the best kind of provender, is unable to fatten, might, after the operation of spaying, be easily fattened, and rendered fit for the market; or, if they shall have had calves, they may be made permanent, and, of course, profitable milkers.

If a cow be in a weak, debilitated state, or, in other words, "out of condition," she may turn out to be a source of great loss to the owner. In the first place, her offspring will be weak and inefficient; successive generations will deteriorate; and if the offspring be in a close degree of relationship, they will scarcely be worth the trouble of rearing. The spaying of such a cow, rather than she shall give birth to weak and worthless offspring, would be a great blessing; for then one of the first causes of degeneracy in live stock will have been removed.

Again, a cow in poor condition is a curse to the farmer; for she is often the medium through which epidemics, infectious diseases, puerperal fever, &c., are communicated to other stock. If there are such diseases in the vicinity, those in poor flesh are sure to be the first victims; and they, coming in contact with others laboring under a temporary indisposition, involve them in the general ruin. If prevention be cheaper than cure, — and who doubts it? — then the farmer should avail himself of the protection which spaying seems to hold out.

OPERATION OF SPAYING.

The first and most important object in the successful performance of this operation is to secure the cow, so that she shall not injure herself, nor lie down, nor be able to kick or injure the operator. The most convenient method of securing the cow is, to place her in the trevis;* the hind legs

* Although we recommend that cows be confined in the trevis for the purpose of performing this operation, it by no means follows that it cannot be done as well in other ways. In fact, the trevis is inadmissible where chloroform is used. The animal must be cast in order to use that agent with any degree of safety. If the trevis is not at hand, we should prefer to operate, having the cow secured to the floor, or held in that position by trusty assistants. We lately operated on a cow, the property of Mr. C

should then be securely tied in the usual manner: the band used for the purpose of raising the hind quarters when being shod must be passed under the belly, and tightened just sufficient to prevent the animal lying down. Having secured the band in this position, we proceed, with the aid of two or more assistants, in case the animal should be irritable, to perform the operation. And here, for the benefit of that portion of our readers who desire to perform the operation *secundum artem*, we detail the method recommended by Morin, a French veterinary surgeon; although it has been, and can again be, performed with a common knife, a curved needle, and a few silken threads to close the external wound. The author is acquainted with a farmer, now a resident of East Boston, who has performed this operation with remarkable success, both in

Drake of Holliston, in this state, under very unfavorable circumstances; yet, as will appear from the accompanying note, the cow is likely to do well, notwithstanding. The history of the case is as follows: We were sent for by Mr. D. to see a heifer having a swelling under the jaw, which proved to be a scirrhous gland. After giving our opinion and prescribing the usual remedies, the conversation turned upon spaying cattle; and Mr. D. remarked that he had a five year old cow, on which we might, if we chose, operate This we rather objected to at first, as the cow was in a state of plethora, and the stomach very much distended with food; yet, as the owner appeared willing to share the responsibility, we consented to perform the operation. The cow was accordingly cast, in the usual manner, she lying on her right side, her head being firmly held by an assistant. We then made an incision through the skin, muscles, and peritoneum. The hand was then introduced, and each ovary in its turn brought as near to the external wound as possible, and separated from its attachment with a button-pointed bistoury. The wound was then brought together with four interrupted sutures, and dressed as already described. Directions were given to keep the animal quiet, and on a light diet; the calf, which was four weeks old, to suckle as usual. The operation was performed on the 17th of January, 1851, and on the 27th, the following communication was received:—

DR. DADD.

Dear Sir: Agreeably to request, I will inform you as regards the cow. I must say that, so far as appearances are concerned, she is doing well. She has a good appetite, and chews her cud, and the wound is not swelled or inflamed. Yours truly, C. DRAKE.

HOLLISTON, *Jan.* 27, 1851.

this country and Scotland, with no other instruments than a common shoemaker's knife and a curved needle. The fact is, the ultimate success of the operation does not depend so much on the instruments as on the skill of the operator. If he is an experienced man, understands the anatomy of the parts, and is well acquainted, by actual experience, with the nature of the operation, then the instruments become a matter of taste. The best operators are those who devote themselves entirely to the occupation. (See Mr. Blane's account of his "first essay in firing," p. 85, note.) Morin advises us to secure the cow, by means of five rings, to the wall. (See Albany Cultivator, vol. vi. p. 244, 1850.) "The cow being conveniently disposed of, and the instruments and appliances, - such as curved scissors, upon a table, a convex-edged bistoury, a straight one, and one buttoned at the point, suture needle filled with double thread of desired length, pledgets of lint of appropriate size and length, a mass of tow (in pledgets) being collected in a shallow basket, held by an assistant,— we place ourselves opposite to the left flank, our back turned a little towards the head of the animal; we cut off the hair which covers the hide in the middle of the flanks, at an equal distance between the back and hip, for the space of thirteen or fourteen centimetres in circumference; this done, we take the convex bistoury, and place it open between our teeth, the edge out, the point to the left; then, with both hands, we seize the hide in the middle of the flank, and form of it a wrinkle of the requisite elevation, and running lengthwise of the body.

"We then direct an assistant to seize, with his right hand, the right side of this wrinkle. We then take the bistoury, and cut the wrinkle at one stroke through the middle: the wrinkle having been suffered to go down, a separation of the hide is presented of sufficient length to enable us to introduce the hand; thereupon we separate the edges of the hide with the thumb and fore finger of the left hand, and, in like manner, we cut through the abdominal muscles, the iliac, (rather obliquely,) and the lumbar, (cross,) for a distance of a centimetre from the lower extremity of the incision made in the hide: this done, armed with the straight bistoury, we make a puncture of the peritoneum, at the upper extremity of the wound; we then introduce the buttoned bistoury, and we move it obliquely from above to the lower part up to the termination of the incision made in the abdominal muscles. The flank being opened, we introduce the right hand into the abdomen, and direct it along the right side of the cavity of the pelvis, behind the paunch and underneath the rectum, where we find the horns of the uterus; after we have ascertained the position of these viscera, we search for the ovaries, which are at the extremity of the *cornua*, or horns, (fallopian tubes,) and when we have found them, we seize them between the thumb and fore finger, detach them completely from the ligaments that keep them in their place, pull lightly, separating the cord, and the vessels (uterine or fallopian tubes) at their place of union with the ovarium, by means of the nails of the thumb and fore finger, which presents itself at the point of touch; in fact, we break the cord, and bring away the ovarium.

"We then introduce again the hand in the abdominal cavity, and we proceed in the same manner to extract the other ovarium.

"This operation terminated, we, by the assistance of a needle, place a suture of three or four double threads, waxed, at an equal distance, and at two centimetres, or a little less, from the lips of the wound; passing it through the divided tissues, we move from the left hand with the piece of thread; having reached that point, we fasten with a double knot; we place the seam in the intervals of the thread from the right, and as we approach the lips of the wound, we fasten by a simple knot, being careful not to close too tightly the lower part of the seam, so that the suppuration, which may be established in the wound, may be able to escape.

"The operation effected, we cover up the wound with a pledget of lint, kept in its place by three or four threads passed through the stitches, and all is completed

"It happens, sometimes, that in cutting the muscles of which we have before spoken, we cut one or two of the arteries, which bleed so much that there is necessity for a ligature before opening the peritoneal sac, because, if this precaution be omitted, blood will escape into the abdomen, and may occasion the most serious consequences."

The best time for spaying cows, with a view of making them permanent milkers, is between the ages of five and seven, especially if they have had two or three calves. If intended to be fattened for beef, the operation should not be performed until the animal has passed its second year, nor after the twelfth.

We usually prepare the animal by allowing a scalded mash every night, within a few days of the operation. The same precaution is observed after the operation.

If, after the operation, the animal appears dull and irritable and refuses her food, the following drink must be given: —

Valerian, ...	2 ounces.
Boiling water, ...	2 quarts.

Set the mixture aside to cool. Then strain, and add infusion of marshmallows (see APPENDIX) one quart; which may be given in pint doses every two hours.

If a bad discharge sets up from the wound, — but this will seldom happen, unless the system abounds in morbific materials, — then, in addition to the drink, wash the wound with

Pyroligneous acid, ...	2 ounces.
Water, ...	2 quarts.

Mix.

SHEEP.

PRELIMINARY REMARKS.

MANY of the diseases to which sheep are subject can be traced to want of due care in their management. The common practice of letting them range in marshy lands is one of the principal causes of disease.

The feet of sheep are organized in such a manner as to be capable, when in a healthy state, of eliminating from the system a large amount of worn-out materials — excrementitious matter, which, if retained in the system, would be injurious. The direct application of cold tends to contract the mouths of excrementitious vessels, and the morbid matter accumulates. This is not all. There are in the system numerous outlets, — for example, the kidneys, lungs, surface, feet, &c. The health of the animal depends on all these functions being duly performed. If a certain function be interrupted for any length of time, it is sure to derange the system. Diseases of the feet are very common in wet situations, and are a source of great loss to the farming community. Hence it becomes a matter of great importance to know how to manage them so as to prevent diseases of the feet.

Professor Simonds says, "No malady was probably so much feared by the agriculturist as the rot; and with reason, for it was most destructive to his hopes. It was commonly believed to be incurable, and therefore it was all important to inquire into the causes which gave rise to it. Some pastures were notorious for rotting sheep; on other lands, sheep, under all ordinary circumstances, were pastured with impunity; but, as a broad principle, it might be laid down that an excess of moisture is prejudicial to the health of the animal. Sheep, by nature, are not only erratic animals, wandering over a large space of ground, but are also inhabitants of arid districts. The skill of man has increased and improved the breed, and has naturalized the animal in moist and temperate climates. But, nevertheless, circumstances now and then take place which show that its nature is not entirely changed; thus, a wet season occurs, the animals are exposed to the debilitating effects of moisture, and the rot spreads among them to a fearful extent. The malady is not confined to England or to Europe; it is found in Asia and Africa, and occurs also in Egypt on the receding of the waters of the Nile.

"These facts are valuable, because they show that the cause of the disease is not local — that it is not produced by climate or temperature; for it is found that animals in any temperature become affected, and on any soil in certain seasons. A great deal had been written on rot in sheep, which it were to be wished had not been. Many talented individuals had devoted their time to its investigation, endeavoring to trace out a cause for it, as if it originated from one cause alone. But the facts here alluded to would show that it arose from more causes than one. He had mentioned the circumstance with regard to land sometimes producing rot. and sometimes not; but he would go a step further, and ask, Was there any particular period of the year when animals were more subject to the attack? Undoubtedly there was. In the rainy season, the heat and moisture combined would produce a most luxuriant herbage; but that herbage would be deficient in nutriment, and danger would be run; the large quantity of watery matter in the food acting as a direct excitement to the abnormal functions of the digestive organs. Early disturbance of the liver led to the accumulation of fat, (state of plethora;) consequently, an animal being 'touched with the rot' thrived much more than usual. This reminded him that the celebrated Bakewell was said to be in the habit of placing his sheep on land notorious for rotting them, in order to prevent other people from getting his stock, and likewise to bring them earlier to market for the butcher."

Referring to diseases of the liver, Professor S. remarked, that "the bile in rot, in consequence of the derangement of the liver being continued, lost the property of converting the chymous mass into nutritious matter, and the animal fell away in condition. Every part of the system was now supplied with impure blood, for we might as well expect pure water from a poisoned fountain as pure blood when the secretion of bile was unhealthy. This state of the liver and the system was associated with the existence of parasites in the liver.

"Some persons suppose that these parasites, which, from their particular form, were called flukes, were the cause of the rot. They are only the effect; yet it is to be remembered that they multiply so rapidly that they become the cause of further diseased action. Sheep, in the earlier stages of the affection, before their biliary ducts become filled with flukes, may be restored; but, when the parasites existed in abundance, there was no chance of the animal's recovery. Those persons who supposed flukes to be the cause of rot had, perhaps, some reason for that opinion. Flukes are oviparous; their ova mingle with the biliary secretion, and thus find their way out of the intestinal canal into the soil; as in the feculent matter of rotten sheep may be found millions of flukes. A Mr. King, of Bath, (England,) had unhesitatingly given it as his opinion that flukes were the cause of rot; believing that, if sheep were pastured on land where the ova existed, they would be taken up with the food, enter into the ramifications of the biliary ducts, and thus contaminate the whole liver. There appeared some ground for this assertion, because very little indeed was known with reference to the duration of life in its latent form in the egg. How long the eggs of birds would remain without undergoing change, if not placed under circumstances favorable to the development of life in a more active form, was undecided. It was the same with the ova of these parasites; so long as they remained on the pasture they underwent no change; but place them in the body of the animal, and subject them to the influence of heat, &c., then those changes would commence which ended in the production of perfect flukes. Take another illustration of the long duration of latent life: Wheat had been locked up for hundreds of years — nay, for thousands — in Egyptian mummies, without undergoing any change, and yet, when planted, had been found prolific.

. . He was not, then, to say that rot was in all cases a curable affection; but at the same time he was fully aware that many animals, that are now considered incurable, might be restored, if sufficient attention was given to them. About two years ago, he purchased seven or eight sheep, all of them giving indisputable proof of rot in its advanced stage. He intended them for experiment and dissection; but as he did not require all of them, and during the winter season only he could dissect, he kept some till summer. They were supplied with food of nutritious quality, free from moisture; they were also protected from all storms and changes of weather, being placed in a shed. The result was, that without any medicine, two of these rotten sheep quite recovered; and when he killed them, although he found that the liver had undergone some change, still the animals would have lived on for years. Rot, in its advanced stage, was a disease which might be considered as analogous to dropsy. A serous fluid accumulates in various parts of the body, chiefly beneath the cellular tissue; consequently, some called it the *water* rot, others the *fluke* rot; but these were merely indications of the same disease in different stages. If flukes were present, it was evident that, in order to strike at the root of the malady, they must get rid of these *entozoa*, and that could only be effected by bringing about a healthy condition of the system. Nothing that could be done by the application of medicine would act on them to affect their vitality. It was only by strengthening their animal powers that they were enabled to give sufficient tone to the system to throw off the flukes: for this purpose many advocated salt. Salt was an excellent stimulative to the digestive organs, and might also be of service in restoring the biliary secretion, from the soda which it contained. So well is its stimulative action known, that some individuals always keep salt in the troughs containing the animal's food. This was a preventive, they had good proof, seeing that it mattered not how moist the soil might be in salt marshes; no sheep were ever attacked by rot in them, whilst those sent there infected very often came back free. Salt, therefore, must not be neglected; but then came the question, Could they not do something more? He believed they could give tonics with advantage. . . . .

"The principles he wished to lay down were, to husband the animals' powers by placing them in a situation where they should not be exposed to the debilitating effects of cold storms; to supply them with nutritious food, and such as contained but a small quantity of water; and, as a stimulant to the digestive organs, to mix it with salt."

The remarks of Professor S. are valuable to the American farmer. First, because they throw some light on the character of a disease but imperfectly understood; secondly, they recommend a safe, efficient, and common-sense method of treating it; and lastly, they recommend such preventive measures as, in this enlightened age, every farmer must acknowledge to be the better part of sheep doctoring. The reader will easily perceive the reason why the food of sheep is injurious when wet or saturated with its own natural juices, when he learns that the digestive process is greatly retarded, unless the masticated food be well saturated with the gastric fluid. If the gastric fluid cannot pervade it, then fermentation takes place; by which process the nutritive properties of the food are partly destroyed, and what remains cannot be taken up before it passes from the vinous into the acetous or putrefactive fermentation; the natural consequence is, that internal disease ensues, which often gravitates to the feet, thereby producing rot. This is not all. Such food does not furnish sufficient material to replenish the daily waste and promote the living integrity. In short, it produces debility, and debility includes one half the causes of disease. It must be a matter of deep interest to the farmer to know how to prevent disease in his flock, and improve their condition, &c.; for if he possessed the requisite knowledge, he would not be compelled to offer mutton at so low a rate as from three to four cents a pound, at which price it is often sold in the Boston market. We have already alluded to the fact that neat cattle can, with the requisite knowledge, be improved at least twenty-five per cent.; and we may add, without fear of contradiction, that the same applies to sheep. If, then, their value can be increased in the same ratio as that of other classes of live stock, how much will the proprietors of sheep gain by the operation? Suppose we set down the number of sheep in the United States at twenty-seven millions, — which will not fall far short of the mark, — and value them at the low price of one dollar per head: we get a clear gain, in the carcasses alone, of six millions seven hundred and fifty thousand dollars. The increase in the quantity, and of course in the value, of wool would pay the additional expenses incurred. It is a well-known fact that, when General Washington left his estate to engage in the councils of his country, his sheep then yielded five pounds of wool. At the time of his return, the animals had so degenerated as to yield but two and a half pounds per fleece. This was not altogether owing to the quality of their food, but in part to want of due care in breeding.

It is well known that many diseases are propagated and aggravated through the sexual congress; and no matter how healthy the dam is, or how much vital resistance she possesses, — if the male be weak and diseased, the offspring will be more or less diseased at birth. (See article *Breeding*.)

Dr. Whitlaw observes, "The Deity has given power to man to ameliorate his condition, as may be truly seen by strict attention to the laws of nature. An attentive observer may soon perceive, that milk, butter, and meat, of animals that feed on good herbage, in high and dry soils, are the best; and that strong nourishment is the produce of those animals that feed on bottom land; but those that feed on a marshy, wet soil produce more acrid food, even admitting that the herbage be of the bland and nutritious kind; but if it be composed in part of poisonous plants, the sheep become diseased and rotten, much more so than cattle, for they do not drink to the same degree, and therefore (particularly those that chew the cud) are not likely to throw off the poison. Horses would be more liable to disease than cattle were it not for their sagacity in selecting the wholesome from the poisonous herbage.

"A great portion of the mutton slaughtered is unfit for food, from the fact that their lungs are often in a state of decomposition, their livers much injured by insects, and their intestines in a state of ulceration, from eating poisonous herbs."

Linnæus says, "A dry place renders plants sapid; a succulent place, insipid; and a watery place, corrosive."

One farmer, in the vicinity of Sherburne, (England,) had, during the space of a few weeks, lost nearly nine hundred sheep by the rot. The fear of purchasing diseased mutton is so prevalent in families, that the demand for mutton has become extremely limited.

In the December number of the London Veterinarian we find an interesting communication from the pen of Mr. Tavistock, V. S., which will throw some light on the causes of disease in sheep. The substance of these remarks is as follows: "On a large farm, situated in the fertile valley of the Tavey, is kept a large flock of sheep, choice and well bred. It is deemed an excellent sheep farm, and for some years no sheep could be healthier than were his flock. About eighteen months ago, however, some ewes were now and then found dead. This was attributed to some of the many maladies sheep-flesh is 'heir to,' and thought no more about. Still it did not cease; another and another died, from time to time, until at length, it becoming a question of serious consequence, my attention was called to them. I made, as opportunities occurred, minute post mortem examinations. The sheep did not die rapidly, but one a week, and sometimes one a fortnight, or even three weeks. No previous illness whatever was manifested. They were always found dead in the attitude of sleep; the countenance being tranquil and composed, not a blade of grass disturbed by struggling; nor did any circumstance evidence that pain or suffering was endured. It was evident that the death was sudden. We fancied the ewes must obtain something poisonous from the herbage, and the only place they could get any thing different from the other sheep was in the orchards, since there the ewes went at the lambing time, and occasionally through the summer. But so they had done for years before, and yet contracted no disease. Well, then, the orchards were the suspected spots, and it was deemed expedient to request Mr. Bartlett, a botanist, to make a careful examination of the orchards, and give us his opinion thereon. The following is the substance of his report: —

"The part of the estate to which the sheep unfortunately had access, where the predisposing causes of disease prevailed, was an orchard, having a gradual slope of about three quarters of a mile in extent, from the high ground to the bed of the river, ranging about east and west; the hills on each side being constituted of argillaceous strata of laminated slate, which, although having an angle of inclination favoring drainage on the slopes, yet in the valleys often became flat or horizontal, and on which also accumulated the clays, and masses of rock, in detached blocks, often to the depth of twenty feet — a state of things which gives the valley surface and soil a very rugged and unequal outline; the whole, at the same time, offering the greatest obstruction to regular drainage.

"These are spots selected for orchard draining in England; the truth being lost sight of, that surfaces and soil for apple-tree growth require the most perfect admixture with atmospheric elements, and the freest outlet for the otherwise accumulating moisture, to prevent dampness and acidity, the result of the shade of the tree itself, produced by the fall of the leaf.

"On this estate these things had never been dreamt of before planting the orchards. The apple-tree, in short, as soon as its branches and leaves spread with the morbid growth of a dozen years, aids itself in the destructive process; the soil becomes yearly more poisonous, the roots soon decay, and the tree falls to one side, as we witness daily, while the herbage beneath and around becomes daily more unfit to sustain animal life. Numerous forms of poisonous fungi, microscopic and otherwise, are here at home, and nourished by the carburetted and other forms of hydrogen gas hourly engendered and saturating the soil; while on the dampest spots the less noxious portions of such hydrates are assimilated by the mint plant in the shape of oil; and which disputes with sour, poisonous, and blossomless grasses for the occupancy of the surface, mingled with the still more noxious straggling forms of the ethusa, occasionally the angelica, vison, conium, &c.

"This state of things, brought into existence by this wretched and barbarous mode of planting orchard valleys, usually reaches its consummation in about thirty years, and sometimes much less, as in the valley under notice. Thus it is that such spots, often the richest in capabilities on the estate, (the deep soil being the waste and spoil of the higher ground and slopes,) become a bane to every form of useful vegetation; and, at the same time, are a hotbed of luxuriance to every thing that is poisonous, destructive, and deleterious to almost every form of animal life. And such an animal as the sheep, while feeding among such herbage, would inhale a sufficiency of noxious gases, especially in summer, through the nostrils alone, to produce disease even in a few hours, though the herbage devoured should lie harmless in the stomach. But with regard to the sheep in the present case, we fear they had no choice in the matter, and were driven by hunger to feed, being shut into these orchards; and thus not only ate the poisoned grasses, but with every mouthful swallowed a portion of the water-engendering mint, the acrid crowfoot, ranunculus leaves, &c., surrounding every blade of grass; while the other essential elements of vegetable poison, the most virulent forms of agarici and their spawn, with other destructive fungi, were swallowed as a sauce to the whole

This fearful state of things, to which sheep had access, soon manifested its results; for although a hog or a badger might here fatten, yet to an animal so susceptible to atmospheric influences, unwholesome, undrained land, &c., as the sheep, the organization forbids the assimilation of such food; and although a process of digestion goes on, yet its hydrous results (if we may use such a term) not only overcharge the blood with serum, but, through unnatural channels, cause effusion into the chest, heart, veins, &c., when its effects are soon manifested in sudden and quick dissolution, being found dead in the attitude of sleep."

It is probable that the gases which arose from this imperfectly drained estate played their part in the work of destruction; not only by coming in immediate contact with the blood through the medium of the air-cells in the lungs, but by mixing with the food in the process of digestion. This may appear a new idea to those who have never given the subject a thought; yet it is no less true. During the mastication of food, the saliva possesses the remarkable property of enclosing air within its globules. Professor Liebig tells us that "the saliva encloses air in the shape of froth, in a far higher degree than even soap-suds. This air, by means of the saliva, reaches the stomach with the food, and there its oxygen enters into combination, while its nitrogen is given out through the skin and lungs." This applies to pure air. Now, suppose the sheep are feeding in pastures notorious for giving out noxious gases, and at the same time the function of the skin or lungs is impaired; instead of the "nitrogen" or noxious gases being set free, they will accumulate in the alimentary canal and cellular tissues, to the certain destruction of the living integrity. Prof. L. further informs us that "the longer digestion continues, — that is, the greater resistance offered to the solvent action by the food, — the more saliva, and consequently the more air, enter the stomach."

STAGGERS.

This disease is known to have its origin in functional derangement of the stomach; and owing to the sympathy that exists between the brain and the latter, derangements are often overlooked, until they manifest themselves by the animal's appearing dull and stupid, and separating itself from the rest of the flock. An animal attacked with staggers is observed to go round in a giddy manner; the optic nerve becomes paralyzed, and the animal often appears blind. It sometimes continues to feed well until it dies.

Indications of Cure. — First, to remove the cause. If it exist in a too generous supply of food, reduce the quantity. If, on the other hand, the animal be in poor condition, a generous supply of nutritious food must be allowed.

Secondly, to impart healthy action to the digestive organs, and lubricate their surfaces.

Having removed the cause, take

Powdered	snakeroot, ...	1 ounce.
"	slippery elm, . . .	2 ounces.
"	fennel seed, ...	half an ounce.

Mix. Half a table-spoonful may be given daily in warm water, or it may be mixed in the food.

Another.

Powdered	gentian, ...	1 ounce.
"	poplar bark, ...	2 ounces.
"	aniseed, ...	half an ounce.

Mix, and give as above.

If the bowels are inactive, give a wine-glass of linseed oil.

The animal should be kept free from all annoyance by dogs, &c.; for fear indirectly influences the stomach through the pneumogastric nerves, by which the secretion of the gastric juice is arrested, and an immediate check is thus given to the process of digestion. For the same reason, medicine should always be given in the food, if possible. In cases of great prostration, accompanied with loss of appetite, much valuable time would be lost. In such cases, we must have recourse to the bottle.

FOOT ROT.

When a sheep is observed to be lame, and, upon examination, matter can be discovered, then pare away the hoof, and make a slight puncture, so that the matter may escape; then wash the foot with the following antiseptic lotion:—

Pyroligneous acid, ...	2 ounces.
Water, ...	3 ounces.

Suppose that, on examination, the feet have a fetid odor; then apply the following:—

Vinegar, ...	half a pint.
Common salt, ...	1 table-spoonful.
Water, ...	half a pint.

Mix, and apply daily. At the same time, put the sheep in a dry place, and give a dose of the following every morning:—

Powdered bayberry bark, . .	half an ounce.
" flaxseed, ...	2 pounds.
" sulphur, ...	1 ounce.
" charcoal, ...	1 ounce.
" sassafras, ...	1 ounce.

Mix. A handful to be given in the food twice a day.

Remarks.—Foot rot is generally considered a local disease; yet should it be neglected, or maltreated, the general system will share in the local derangement.

ROT.

The progress of this disease is generally very slow, and a person unaccustomed to the management of sheep would find some difficulty in recognizing it. A practical eye would distinguish it, even at a distance. The disease is known by one or more of the following symptoms: The animal often remains behind the flock, shaking its head, with its ears depressed; it allows itself to be seized, without any resistance. The eye is dull and watery; the eyelids are swollen; the lips, gums, and palate have a pale tint; the skin, which is of a yellowish white, appears puffed, and retains the impression; the wool loses its brightness, and is easily torn off; the urine is high colored, and the excrement soft. As the disease progresses, there is loss of appetite, great thirst, general emaciation, &c.

The indications are, to improve the secretions, vitalize the blood, and sustain the living powers. For which purpose, take

Powdered charcoal, ...	2 ounces.
" ginger, ...	1 ounce.
" golden seal, ...	1 ounce.
Oatmeal, ...	1 pound.

Mix. Feed to each animal a handful per day, unless rumination shall have ceased; then omit the oatmeal, and give a tea-spoonful of the mixed ingredients, in half a pint of hyssop, or horsemint tea. Continue as occasion may require.

The food should be boiled, if possible. The best kind, especially in the latter stages of rot, is, equal parts of linseed and ground corn.

If the urine is high colored, and the animal is thirsty, give an occasional drink of

Cleavers, (*galium aparine,*)	2 ounces.
Boiling water, ...	2 quarts.

When cold, strain. Dose, one pint. To be repeated, if necessary.

EPILEPSY.

This is somewhat different from staggers, as the animal does not remain quietly on the ground, but it suffers from convulsions, it kicks, rolls its eyes, grinds its teeth, &c. The duration of the fit varies much: sometimes it terminates at the expiration of a few minutes; at other times, a quarter of an hour elapses before it is perfectly conscious. In this malady, there is a loss of equilibrium between the nervous and muscular systems, which may arise from hydatids in the brain, offering mechanical obstructions to the conducting power of the nerves. This malady may attack animals in apparently good health. We frequently see children attacked with epilepsy (fits) without any apparent cause, and when they are in good flesh.

The symptoms are not considered dangerous, except by their frequent repetition.

The following may be given with a view of equalizing the circulation and nervous action: —

Assafœtida, ...	one third of a tea-spoonful.
Gruel made from slippery elm,	1 pint.

Mix, while hot. Repeat the dose every other day. Make some change in the food. Thus, if the animal has been fed on green fodder for any length of time, let it have a few meals of shorts, meal, linseed, &c. The water must be of the best quality.

Suppose the animal to be in poor condition; then combine tonics and alteratives in the following form: —

Assafœtida, ...	1 tea-spoonful.
Powdered golden seal, . . .	1 ounce.
" slippery elm, . . .	2 ounces.
Oatmeal, ...	1 pound.

Mix thoroughly, and divide into eight equal parts. A powder to be given every morning.

RED WATER.

This is nothing more nor less than a symptom of deranged function. The cure consists in restoring healthy action to all parts of the animal organization. For example, high-colored urine shows that there is too much action on the internal surfaces, and too little on the external. This at once points to the propriety of keeping the sheep in a warm situation, in order to invite action to the skin.

Compound for Red Water.

Powdered slippery elm, . .	of each, 1 ounce.
" pleurisy root, . .	of each, 1 ounce.
" poplar bark, . .	of each, 1 ounce.
Indian meal, ...	1 pound.

Mix. To be divided into ten parts, one of which may be given every morning.

CACHEXY,* OR GENERAL DEBILITY.

Indications of Cure. — First. To build up and promote the living integrity by a generous diet, one or more of the following articles may be scalded and given three times a day: carrots, parsnips, linseed, corn meal, &c.

Secondly. To remove morbific materials from the system, and restore the lost functions, one of the following powders may be given, night and morning, in the fodder: —

Powdered balmony, (snakehead,) .	1 ounce.
" marshmallows, . . .	1 ounce.
" common salt, ...	1 table-spoonful.
Linseed meal, ...	1 pound.

Mix. Divide into ten powders.

LOSS OF APPETITE.

This is generally owing to a morbid state of the digestive organs. All that is necessary in such case is, to restore the lost tone by the exhibition of bitter tonics. A bountiful supply of camomile tea will generally prove sufficient. If, however, the bowels are inactive, add to the above a small portion of extract of butternut. The food should be slightly salted.

FOUNDERING, (RHEUMATISM.)

In this malady, the animal becomes slow in its movements· its walk is characterized by rigidity of the muscular

* It implies a vitiated state of the solids and fluids.

system, and, when lying down, requires great efforts in order to rise.

Causes. — Exposure to sudden changes in temperature, feeding on wet lands, &c.

Indications of Cure. — To equalize the circulation, invite and maintain action to the external surface, and remove the cause. To fulfil the latter indication, remove the animal to a dry, warm situation.

The following antispasmodic and diaphoretic will complete the cure: Powdered lady's slipper, (*cypripedium*,) 1 tea-spoonful. To be given every morning in a pint of warm pennyroyal tea.

If the malady does not yield in a few days, take

Powdered sassafras bark, . . .	1 tea-spoonful.
Boiling water, ...	1 pint.
Honey, ...	1 tea-spoonful.

Mix, and repeat the dose every other morning.

TICKS.

Ticks, or, in short, any kind of insects, may be destroyed by dropping on them a few drops of an infusion or tincture of lobelia seeds.

SCAB, OR ITCH.

Scab, itch, erysipelas, &c., all come under the head of cutaneous diseases, and require nearly the same general treatment. The following compound may be depended on as a safe and efficient remedy in either of the above diseases: —

Sulphur, ...	2 ounces.
Powdered sassafras, ...	1 ounce.

Honey, sufficient to amalgamate the above. Dose, a table-spoonful every morning. To prevent the sheep from rubbing themselves, apply

Pyroligneous acid, ...	1 gill.
Water, ...	1 quart.

Mix, and wet the parts with a sponge.

Remarks. — In reference to the scab, Dr. Gunther says, "Of all the preservatives which have been proposed, inoculation is the best. It has two advantages: first, the disease so occasioned is much more mitigated, and very rarely proves fatal; in the next place, an entire flock may get well from it in the space of fifteen days, whilst the natural form of the disorder requires care and attention for at least six months. It has been ascertained that the latter kills * more than one half of those attacked; whilst among the sheep that have been inoculated, the greatest proportion that die of it is one per cent."

Whenever the scab makes its appearance, the whole flock should be examined, and every one having the least abrasion or eruption of the skin should be put under medical treatment.

In most cases, itch is the result of infection. A single sheep infected with it is sufficient to infect a whole flock. If a few applications of the pyroligneous wash, aided by the medicine, are not sufficient to remove the malady, then recourse must be had to the following: —

Fir balsam, ...	half a pint.
Sulphur, ...	1 ounce.

Mix. Anoint the sores daily.

* More likely the remedies. They are tobacco and corrosive sublimate

The only additional treatment necessary in erysipelas is, to give a bountiful supply of tea made of lemon balm, sweetened with honey.

DIARRHŒA.

This is not always to be considered as a disease, but in many cases it proves a salutary operation of nature; therefore it should not be too suddenly checked.

We commence the treatment by feeding on boiled meal. We then give mucilaginous drink made from marshmallows, slippery elm, or poplar bark. If, at the end of two days, symptoms of amendment have not made their appearance the following draught must be given: —

Make a strong infusion of raspberry leaves, to a pint of which add a tea-spoonful of tincture of capsicum, (hot drops,) and one of charcoal. To be repeated every morning, until healthy action is established.

DYSENTERY.

This malady may be treated in the same manner as diarrhœa. Should blood and slime be voided in large quantities, the excrement emit a fetid odor, and the animal waste rapidly, then, in addition to the mucilaginous drink, administer the following: —

Powdered charcoal,	. . . . .	1 tea-spoonful.
" golden seal,	. . . .	half a tea-spoonful.

To be given, in hardhack tea, as occasion may require.

A small quantity of charcoal, given three times a day, with boiled food, will frequently cure the disease, alone.

Dysentery is sometimes mistaken for diarrhœa; but they may be distinguished by the following characteristics: —

1st. Diarrhœa most frequently attacks weak animals; whereas dysentery ofttimes attacks animals in good condition.

2d. Dysentery generally attacks sheep in the hot months; on the other hand, diarrhœa terminates at the commencement of the hot season.

3d. In diarrhœa, there are scarcely any feverish symptoms, and no straining before evacuation, as in dysentery.

4th. In diarrhœa, the excrement is loose, but in other respects natural, without any blood or slime; whereas in dysentery the fæces consist of hard lumps, blood, and slime.

5th. There is not that degree of fetor in the fæces, in diarrhœa, which takes place in dysentery.

6th. In dysentery, the appetite is totally gone; in diarrhœa, it is generally better than usual.

7th. Diarrhœa is not contagious; dysentery is supposed to be highly so.

8th. In dysentery, the animal wastes rapidly; but by diarrhœa, only a temporary stop is put to thriving, after which it makes rapid advances to strength, vigor, and proportion.

CONSTIPATION, OR STRETCHES.

By these terms are implied a preternatural or morbid detention and hardening of the excrement; a disease to which all animals are subject, unless proper attention be paid to their management. It mostly arises from want of exercise, feeding on frosted oats, indigestible matter of every kind, impure water, &c. Costiveness is often the cause of flatulent and spasmodic colic, and often of inflammation of the bowels.

Mr. Morrill says, "I have always found that the quantity of medicine necessary to act as an *opiate* on this dry mass [alluding to that found in the manyplus and intestines] will kill the animal. If I am mistaken, I will take it kindly to be set right." You are quite right.

Let us see what Professor J. A. Gallup says, in his Institutes of Medicine, vol. ii. p. 187. "The practice of giving opiates to mitigate pain, &c., is greatly to be deprecated; it is not only unjustifiable, but should be esteemed unpardonable. It is probable that, for forty years past, opium and its preparations have done *seven times the injury* that they have rendered benefit" — killed seven where they have saved one! Page 298, he calls opium the "most destructive of all narcotics," and wishes he could "speak through a lengthened trumpet, that he might tingle the ears" of those who use and prescribe it. All the opiates used by the allopathists contain more or less of this poisonous drug. Opiates given with a view of softening the mass alluded to will certainly disappoint those who administer them; for, under the use of such "palliatives," the digestive powers fail, and a general state of feebleness and inactivity ensues, which exhausts the vital energies.

It will be found in stretches, that other organs, as well as the "manyplus," are not performing their part in the business of physiological or healthy action, and they must be excited to perform their work; for example, if the food remains in either of the stomachs in the form of a hard mass, then the surface of the body is evaporating too much moisture from the general system; the skin should be better toned. Pure air is one of the best and most valuable of nature's tonics. Let the flock have pure air to breathe, and sufficient room to use their limbs, with proper diet, and there will be little occasion for medicine.

Treatment. — The disease is to be obviated by proper attention to diet, exercise, and ventilation; and when these fail, to have recourse to bitter laxatives, injections, and aperients. The use of salts and castor oil creates a necessity for their repetition, for they overwork the mucous surfaces, and their delicate vessels lose their natural sensibility, and become torpid. Scalded shorts are exceedingly valuable in this complaint, as also are boiled carrots, parsnips, &c.

The derangement must be treated according to its indications, thus:—

Suppose the digestive organs to be deranged, and rumination to have ceased; then take a tea-spoonful of extract of butternut, and dissolve it in a pint of thoroughwort tea, and give it at a dose. Use an injection of soap-suds, if necessary.

Suppose the excrement to be hard, coated with slime, and there be danger of inflammation in the mucous surfaces; then give a wine-glass of linseed oil,* to which add a raw egg.

It is scarcely ever necessary to repeat the dose, provided the animal is allowed a few scalded shorts.

If the liver is supposed to be inactive, give, daily, a tea-spoonful of golden seal in the food.

If the animal void worms with the fæces, then give a tea made from cedar boughs, or buds, to which add a small quantity of salt.

SCOURS.

In scours, the surface evaporates too little of the moisture, and should be relaxed by diffusible stimulants in the form of ginger tea. The treatment that we have found the most successful is as follows: take four ounces raw linseed oil, two ounces of lime water; mix. Let this quantity be given to a sheep on the first appearance of the above disease; half the quantity will suffice for a lamb. Give about a wine-glass full of ginger tea at intervals of four hours, or mix a small quantity of ginger in the food. Let the animal be fed on gruel, or mashes of ground meal. If the above treatment fails to arrest the disease, add half a tea-spoonful of powdered bay-

* Olive oil will answer the same purpose.

berry bark. If the extremities are cold, rub them with the tincture of capsicum.

DIZZINESS.

Mr. Gunther says, "Sheep are often observed to describe eccentric circles for whole hours, then step forwards a pace, then again stop, and turn round again. The older the disease, the more the animal turns, until at length it does it even in a trot. The appetite goes on diminishing, emaciation becomes more and more perceptible, and the state of exhaustion terminates in death. On opening the skull, there are met, either beneath the bones of the cranium, or beneath the dura mater,* or in the brain itself, hydatids varying in number and size, sometimes a single one, often from three to six, the size of which varies: according as these worms occupy the right side or the left, the sheep turns to the right or left; but if they exist on both sides, the turning takes place to the one and the other alternately.

"The animal very often does not turn, which happens when the worm is placed on the median line; then the affected animal carries the head down, and though it seems to move rapidly, it does not change place. When the hydatid is situated on the posterior part of the brain, the animal carries the head high, runs straight forward, and throws itself on every object it meets."

Treatment. — Take

Powdered worm seeds, (*chenopodium anthelminticum,*) . . .	1 ounce.
" sulphur, ...	half an ounce
" charcoal, ...	2 ounces.
Linseed, or flaxseed, ...	1 pound.

* The membrane which lines the interior of the skull.

Mix. Divide into eight parts, and feed one every morning. Make a drink from the white Indian hemp, (*asclepias incarnata,*) one ounce of which may be infused in a quart of water, one fourth to be given every night.

JAUNDICE.

This malady generally involves the whole system in its deranged action. It is recognized by the yellow tint of the conjunctiva, (white of the eye,) and mucous membranes lining the nostrils and mouth. We generally employ for its cure

Powdered mandrake,	. . . .	1 tea-spoonful.
" ginger,	. . . . .	1 tea-spoonful.
" golden seal,	. . .	2 tea-spoonfuls.

Mix. Divide into two parts. Give one dose in the morning, and the other at night. An occasional drink of camomile tea, a few bran mashes, and boiled carrots, will complete the cure.

INFLAMMATION OF THE KIDNEYS.

A derangement of these organs may result from external violence, or it may depend on the animal having eaten stimulating or poisonous plants.

Its symptoms are, pain in the region of the kidneys; the back is arched, and the walk stiff and painful, with the legs widely separated; there is a frequent desire to make water, and that is high colored or bloody; the appetite is more or less impaired, and there is considerable thirst.

The indications are, to lubricate the mucous surfaces, remove morbific materials from the system, and improve the general health.

We commence the treatment by giving

Poplar bark, finely powdered, . .	1 ounce.
Pleurisy root, " " . .	1 tea-spoonful.

Make a mucilage of the poplar bark, by stirring in boiling water; then add the pleurisy root; the whole to be given in the course of twenty-four hours. The diet should consist of a mixture of linseed, boiled carrots, and meal.

WORMS.

The intestinal worms generally arise from impaired digestion. The symptoms are, a diminution of rumination, wasting away of the body, and frequent snorting, obstruction of the nostrils with mucus of a greater or less thickness.

Compound for Worms.

Powdered worm seed, ...	equal parts.
" skunk cabbage, . . .	
" ginger, ...	

Dose, a tea-spoonful night and morning in the fodder.

DISEASES OF THE STOMACH FROM EATING POISONOUS PLANTS.

Treatment. — Take the animal from pasture, and put it on a boiled diet, of shorts, meal, linseed, and carrots. The following alterative may be mixed in the food: —

Powdered marshmallows, ...	1 ounce.
" sassafras bark, ...	2 ounces.
" charcoal, ...	2 ounces.
" licorice, ...	2 ounces.

Dose one table-spoonful every night

SORE NIPPLES.

LAMBS often die of hunger, from their dams refusing them suck. The cause of this is sore nipples, or some tumor in the udder, in which violent pain is excited by the tugging of the lamb. Washing with poplar bark, or anointing the teats with powdered borax and honey, will generally effect a cure.

FRACTURES.

THE mending of a broken bone, though somewhat tedious, is by no means difficult, when the integuments are not torn. Let the limb be gently distended, and the broken ends of the bone placed in contact with each other. A piece of stiff leather, of pasteboard, or of thin shingle, wrapped in a soft rag, is then to be laid along the limb, so that it may extend an inch or two beyond the contiguous part. The splints are then to be secured by a bandage of linen an inch and a half broad. After being firmly rolled up, it should be passed spirally round the leg, taking care that every turn of the bandage overlaps about two thirds of the preceding one. When the inequality of the parts causes the margin to slack, it must be reversed or folded over; that is, its upper margin must become the lower, &c. The bandage should be moderately tight, so as to support the parts without intercepting the circulation, and should be so applied as to press equally on every part. The bandage may be occasionally wet with a mixture of equal parts of vinegar and water.

COMMON CATARRH AND EPIDEMIC INFLUENZA.

The seat of the disease is in the mucous membrane, which is a continuation of the external skin, folded into all the orifices of the body, as the mouth, eyes, nose, ears, lungs, stomach, intestines and bladder; its structure of arterial capillaries, veins, arteries, nerves, &c., is similar to the external skin; its most extensive surfaces are those of the lungs and intestines, the former of which is supposed to be greater than the whole external surface of the body.

The healthy office of this membrane is to furnish from the blood a fluid called mucus, to lubricate its own surface, and protect it from the action of materials taken into the system. The mucous membrane and the external surface of the body seem to be a counterpart of each other, and perform nearly the same offices; hence, if the action of one is suppressed, the other commences the performance of its office; thus a cold which closes the skin immediately stops the perspiration, which is now forced through the mucous membrane, producing the discharge of watery humors, pus intermixed with blood, dry cough, emaciation, &c. There are two varieties of this disease; the first is called *common catarrh*, which proceeds from cold taken in pasture that is not properly drained, also from atmospheric changes; it may also proceed from acrid or other irritating effluvia inhaled in the air, or from poisonous substances taken in the stomach in the form of food. The second variety is called *epidemic influenza*, and is produced by general causes; the attack is sometimes sudden; although of nearly the same nature as the first form, it is more obstinate, and the treatment must be more energetic. It is very difficult to lay down correct rules for the treatment of this malady, under its different forms and stages. The principal object to be kept in view is, to equalize the circulation, remove the irritating causes from the organs affected, and restore the tone of the system.

For this purpose, we make use of the following articles:-

Horehound, (herb,)	1 ounce.
Marshallow, (root,)	1 ounce.
Powdered elecampane, (root,) .	half an ounce.
" licorice, "	half an ounce.
Powdered cayenne, . . .	half a tea-spoonful.
Molasses, ...	2 table-spoonfuls.
Vinegar, ...	2 table-spoonfuls.

Mix, pour on the whole one quart of boiling water, set it aside for two hours, then strain through cotton cloth, and give a table-spoonful night and morning.* If the bowels are constipated, a dose of linseed oil should precede the mixture. No water should be allowed during the treatment.

The following injection may be used: —

Powdered bayberry bark, . .	1 ounce.
" gum arabic, . . .	half an ounce.
Boiling water, ...	1 pint.

Stir occasionally while cooling, and strain as above.

The legs and ears should be briskly rubbed with tincture of capsicum; this latter acts as a counter-irritant, equalizes the circulation, and, entering into the system, gives tone and vigor to the whole animal economy.

CASTRATING LAMBS.

The lambs are first driven into a small enclosure. Select the ewe from the ram lambs, and let the former go. Two assistants are necessary. One catches the lambs; the other is seated on a low bench for the purpose of taking the lamb on his lap, where he holds it by the four legs. The operator,

* This preparation undergoes a process of fermentation in the course of forty-eight hours, and should therefore only be made in sufficient quantities for present use.

having previously supplied himself with a piece of waxed silk and the necessary implements, grasps the scrotum in his left hand. He then makes an incision over the most prominent part of the testicle, through the skin, cellular structure, &c. The testicle escapes from the scrotum. A ligature is now passed around the spermatic artery, and tied, and the cord is severed, bringing the testicle away at one stroke of the knife. As soon as the operation is completed, the animal is released. The evening is the best time for performing the operation, for then the animal remains quiet during the night, and the wound heals kindly.

NATURE OF SHEEP.

"The sheep, though in most countries under the protection and control of man, is not that stupid and contemptible animal that has been represented. Amidst those numerous flocks which range without control on extensive mountains, where they seldom depend upon the aid of man, it will be found to assume a very different character. In those situations, a ram or a wether will boldly attack a single dog, and often come off victorious; but when the danger is more alarming, they have recourse to the collected strength of the whole flock. On such occasions, they draw up into a compact body, placing the young and the females in the centre, while the males take the foremost ranks; keeping close by each other. Thus an armed front is presented to all quarters, and cannot be easily attacked, without danger or destruction to the assailant. In this manner they wait with firmness the approach of the enemy; nor does their courage fail them in the moment of attack; for when the aggressor advances to within a few yards of the line, the rams dart upon him with such impetuosity, as to lay him dead at their feet, unless he save himself by flight. Against the attack of a single dog, when in this situation, they are perfectly secure."

THE RAM.

Mr. Lawson says, "It may be observed that the rams of different breeds of sheep vary greatly in their forms, wools, and fleeces, and other properties; but the following description, by that excellent stock-farmer, Mr. Culley, deserves the attention of the breeder and grazier. According to him, the head of the ram should be fine and small; his nostrils wide and expanded; his eyes prominent, and rather bold or daring; his ears thin; his collar full from his breast and shoulders, but tapering gradually all the way to where the neck and head join, which should be very fine and graceful, being perfectly free from any coarse leather hanging down; the shoulders full, which must, at the same time, join so easy to the collar forward, and chine backward, as to leave not the least hollow in either place; the mutton upon his arm or fore thigh must come quite to the knee; his legs upright, with a clean fine bone, being equally clear from superfluous skin and coarse, hairy wool from the knee and hough downwards; the breast broad and well forward, which will keep his fore legs at a proper width; his girt or chest full and deep, and instead of a hollow between the shoulders, that part by some called the fore flank should be quite full; the back and loins broad, flat, and straight, from which the ribs must rise with a fine circular arch; his belly straight; the quarters long and full, with the mutton quite down to the hough, which should neither stand in nor out; his twist, or junction of the inside of the thighs, deep, wide, and full, which, with the broad breast, will keep his legs open and upright; the whole body covered with a thin pelt, and that with fine, bright, soft wool.

"It is to be observed that the neare any breed of sheep come up to the above description, the nearer they approach towards excellence of form."

LEAPING.

"THE manner of treating rams has lately received a very great improvement. Instead of turning them loose among the ewes at large, as heretofore, and agreeably to universal practice, they are kept apart, in a separate paddock, or small enclosure, with a couple of ewes only each, to make them rest quietly; having the ewes of the flock brought to them singly, and leaping each only once. By this judicious and accurate regulation, a ram is enabled to impregnate near twice the number of ewes he would do if turned loose among them, especially a young ram. In the old practice, sixty or eighty ewes were esteemed the full number for a ram. [Overtaxing the male gives rise to weak and worthless offspring.]

"The period during which the rams are to go with the ewes must be regulated by climate, and the quantity of spring food provided. It is of great importance that lambs should be dropped as early as possible, that they not only be well nursed, but have time to get stout, and able to provide for themselves before the winter sets in. It is also of good advantage to the ewes that they may get into good condition before the rutting season. The ram has been known to live to the age of fifteen years, and begins to procreate at one. When castrated, they are called *wethers;* they then grow sooner fat, and the flesh becomes finer and better flavored."

ARGYLESHIRE BREEDERS.

IN Argyleshire, the principal circumstances attended to by the most intelligent sheep-farmers are these: to stock lightly, which will mend the size of the sheep, with the quantity and quality of the wool, and also render them less subject to diseases; (in all these respects it is allowed, by good judges, tha five hundred sheep, kept well, will return more profit than six hundred kept indifferently;) to select the best lambs, and such as have the finest, closest, and whitest wool, for tups and breeding ewes, and to cut and spay the worst; to get a change of rams frequently, and of breeding ewes occasionally; to put the best tups to the best ewes, which is considered necessary for bringing any breed to perfection; not to tup three-year-old ewes, (which, in bad seasons especially would render the lambs produced by them of little value, as the lambs would not have a sufficiency of milk; and would also tend to lessen the size of the stock;) to keep no rams above three, or at most four years old, nor any breeding ewes above five or six; to separate the rams from the 10th of October, for a month or six weeks, to prevent the lambs from coming too early in the spring; to separate the lambs between the 15th and 25th of June; to have good grass prepared for them; and if they can, to keep them separate, and on good grass all winter, that they may be better attended to, and have the better chance of avoiding disease. A few, whose possessions allow them to do it, keep not only their lambs, but also their wethers, ewes, &c., in separate places, by which every man, having his own charge, can attend to it better than if all were in common; and each kind has its pasture that best suits it.

FATTENING SHEEP.

We are indebted to Mr. Cole, editor of the New England Farmer, for the following article, which is worthy the attention of the reader:—

"Quietude and warmth contribute greatly to the fattening process. This is a fact which has not only been developed by science, but proved by actual practice. The manner in which these agents operate is simple, and easily explained.

Motion increases respiration, and the excess of oxygen, thus taken, requires an increased quantity of carbon, which would otherwise be expended in producing fat. So, likewise, *cold robs the system of animal heat;* to supply which, more oxygen and more carbon must be employed in extra combustion, to restore the diminution of temperature. Nature enforces the restoration of warmth, by causing cold to produce both hunger and a disposition for motion, supplying carbon by the gratification of the former, and oxygen by the indulgence of the latter. The above facts are illustrated by Lord Ducie: —

"One hundred sheep were placed in a shed, and ate twenty pounds of Swedish turnips each per day; whilst another hundred, in the open air, ate twenty-five pounds each; and at that rate for a certain period: the former animals weighed each thirty pounds more than the latter; plainly showing that, to a certain extent, *warmth is a substitute for food.* This was also proved, by the same nobleman, in other experiments, which also illustrated the effect of exercise.

"No. 1. Five sheep were fed in the open air, between the 21st of November and the 1st of December. They consumed ninety pounds of food per day, the temperature being 44°. At the end of this time, they weighed two pounds less than when first exposed.

"No. 2. Five sheep were placed under shelter, and allowed to run at a temperature of 49°. They consumed at first eighty-two pounds, then seventy pounds, and increased in weight twenty-three pounds.

"No. 3. Five sheep were placed in the same shed, but not allowed any exercise. They ate at first sixty-four pounds, then fifty-eight pounds, and increased in weight thirty pounds.

"No. 4. Five sheep were kept in the dark, quiet and covered. They ate thirty-five pounds per day, and increased in weight eight pounds.

"A similar experiment was tried by Mr. Childers, M. P. He states, that eighty Leicester sheep, in the open field, consumed fifty baskets of cut turnips per day, besides oil cake

On putting them in a shed, they were immediately able to consume only thirty baskets, and soon after but twenty-five being only one half the quantity required before; and yet they fattened as rapidly as when eating the largest quantity.

"From these experiments, it appears that the least quantity of food, which is required for fattening, is when animals are kept closely confined in warm shelters; and the greatest quantity when running at large, exposed to all weather. But, although animals will fatten faster for a certain time without exercise than with it, if they are closely confined for any considerable time, and are at the same time full fed, they become, in some measure, feverish; the proportion of fat becomes too large, and the meat is not so palatable and healthy as when they are allowed moderate exercise, in yards or small fields.

"As to the kinds of food which may be used most advantageously in fattening, this will generally depend upon what is raised upon the farm, it being preferable, in most cases, to use the produce of the farm. Sheep prefer beans to almost any other grain; but neither beans nor peas are so fattening as some other grains, and are used most advantageously along with them. Beans, peas, oats, barley, rye, buckwheat, &c., may be used along with Indian corn, or oil cake, or succulent food, making various changes and mixtures, in order to furnish the variety of food which is so much relished by the sheep, and which should ever be attended to by the sheep fattener. This will prevent their being cloyed, and will hasten the fattening process. A variety of food, says Mr Spooner, operates like cookery in the human subject, enabling more sustenance to be taken.

"The quantity of grain or succulent food, which it will be proper to feed, will depend upon the size, age, and condition of the sheep; and judgment must be used in ascertaining how much they can bear. Mr. Childers states that sheep (New Leicester) fed with the addition of half a pint of barley per sheep, per day, half a pound of linseed oil cake, with hay, and a constant supply of salt, became ready for the butcher in ten weeks; the gain of flesh and tallow, thirty-three pounds to forty pounds per head. (One sheep gained fifty-five pounds in twelve weeks.)

"This experiment shows what is about the largest amount of grain which it is necessary or proper to feed to New Leicester sheep, at any time while fattening. The average weight of forty New Leicester wethers, before fattening, was found by Mr. Childers to be one hundred and twenty-eight pounds each. By weighing an average lot of any other kind of sheep, which are to be fattened, and by reference to the table of comparative nutriment of the different kinds of food, a calculation may be readily made, as to the largest amount, which will be necessary for them, of any article of food whatever.

"When sheep are first put up for fattening, they should be sorted, when convenient, so as to put those of the same age, size, and condition, each by themselves, so that each may have a fair chance to obtain its proportion of food, and may be fed the proper length of time.

"They should be fed moderately at first, gradually increasing the quantity to the largest amount, and making the proper changes of food, so as not to cloy them, nor produce acute diseases of the head or intestines, and never feeding so much as to scour them.

"Sheep, when fattening, should not be fed oftener than three times a day, viz., morning, noon, and evening. In the intervals between feeding, they may fill themselves well, and will have time sufficient for rumination and digestion: these processes are interrupted by too frequent feeding. But they should be fed with regularity, both as to the quantity of food and the time when it is given. When convenient, they should have access to water at all times; otherwise a full supply of it should be furnished to them immediately after they have consumed each foddering.

"When sheep become extremely fat, whether purposely or not, it is generally expedient to slaughter them. Permitting animals to become alternately very fat and lean is injurious to all stock. Therefore, if animals are too strongly inclined to fatten at an age when wanted for breeding, their condition as to flesh should be regulated by the quantity and quality of their food or pasture."

IMPROVEMENT IN SHEEP.

No country in the world is better calculated for raising sheep than the United States. The diversity of climate, together with the abundance and variety of the products of the soil, united with the industry and perseverance of the agriculturist, renders this country highly favorable for breeding, maturing, and improving the different kinds of sheep. The American people, taken as a whole, are intellectually stronger than any other nation with the like amount of population, on the face of the globe; consequently they are all-powerful, "for the mind is mightier than the sword." All that we aim at, in these pages, is to turn the current of the American mind to the important subject of improvement in the animal kingdom; to show them the great benefits they will derive from practical experience in the management of all classes of live stock; and, lastly, to show them the value and importance of the veterinary profession, when flourishing under the genial influence of a liberal community. If we can only succeed in arresting the attention of American stock raisers, and they, on the other hand, direct their whole attention to the matter, then, in a few years, America will outshine her more favored European rivals, and feel proud of her improved stock. What the American people have done during the last half century in the improvement of the soil, manufactures, arts, and sciences, is an earnest of what they can do in ameliorating the condition of all classes of live stock, provided they take hold of the subject in good earnest. Let any one who is acquainted with the subject of degeneration, its causes and fatal results, not only in reference to the stock itself, but as regards the pocket of the breeder, and the health of the whole community, — let such a one go into our slaughter-houses and markets, and if he does not see a wide field for improvement, then we will agree to let the subject sink into oblivion. In order to show what a whole community can accomplish when their efforts are directed to one object, let us look on what a single individual, by his own industry and perseverance, has accomplished simply in improving the breed of sheep. The person referred to is Mr. Bakewell. His breeding animals were, in the first place, selected from different breeds. These he crossed with the best to be had. After the cross had been carried to the desired point, he confined his selections to his own herds or flocks. He formed in his mind a standard of perfection for each kind of animals, and to this he constantly endeavored to bring them. That he was eminently successful in the attainment of his object, cannot be denied. He began his farming operations about 1750. In 1760, his rams did not sell for more than two or three guineas per head. From this time he gradually advanced in terms, and in 1770 he let some for twenty-five guineas a head for the season. Marshall states that, in 1786, Bakewell let two thirds of a ram (reserving a third for himself) to two breeders, for a hundred guineas each, the entire services of the ram being rated at three hundred guineas the season. It is also stated that he made that year, by letting rams, more than one thousand pounds.

"In 1789, he made twelve hundred guineas by three '*ram brothers*,' and two thousand guineas from seven, and, from his whole letting, full three thousand guineas. Six or seven other breeders made from five hundred to a thousand guineas each by the same operation. The whole amount of ram-letting of Bakewell's breed is said to have been not less, that year, than ten thousand pounds, [forty-eight thousand dollars.]

"It is true that still more extraordinary prices were obtained for the use of rams of this breed after Mr. Bakewell's death. Pitt, in his 'Survey of Leicestershire,' mentions that, in 1795, Mr Astley gave three hundred guineas for the use of a ram of this breed, engaging, at the same time, that he should serve *gratis* twenty ewes owned by the man of whom the ram was hired; making for the entire use of the ram, that season, four hundred and twenty guineas. In 1796, Mr. Astley gave for the use of the same ram three hundred guineas, and took forty ewes to be served gratis. At the price charged for the service of the ram to each ewe, the whole value for the season was five hundred guineas. He served one hundred ewes. In 1797, the same ram was let to another person at three hundred guineas, and twenty ewes sent with him; the serving of which was reckoned at a hundred guineas, and the ram was restricted to sixty more, which brought his value for the season to four hundred guineas. Thus the ram made, in three seasons, the enormous sum of *thirteen hundred guineas.*

"We have nothing to do, at present, with the question whether the value of these animals was not exaggerated. The actual superiority of the breed over the stock of the country must have been obvious, and this point we wish kept in mind.

"This breed of sheep is continued to the present day, and it has been remarked by a respected writer, that they will 'remain a lasting monument of Bakewell's skill.' As to their origin, the testimony shows them to have been of *mixed blood;* though no breed is more distinct in its characters, or transmits its qualities with more certainty; and if we were without any other example of successful crossing, the advocates of the system might still point triumphantly to the Leicester or Bakewell sheep.

"But what are the opinions of our best modern breeders in regard to the practicability of producing distinct breeds by crossing? Robert Smith, of Burley, Rutlandshire, an eminent sheep-breeder, in an essay on the 'Breeding and Managemen of Sheep,' for which he received a prize from the Royal Agricultural Society, (1847,) makes the following remarks: 'The crossing of pure breeds has been a subject of great interest amongst every class of breeders. While all agree that the first cross may be attended with good results, there exists a diversity of opinion upon the future movements, or putting the crosses together. Having tried experiments (and I am now pursuing them for confirmation) in every way possible, I do not hesitate to express my opinion, that, by proper and judicious crossing through several generations, a most valuable breed of sheep may be raised and established; in support of which I may mention the career of the celebrated Bakewell, who raised a *new* variety from other long-wooled breeds by dint of perseverance and propagation, and which have subsequently corrected all other long-wooled breeds.' "

We have alluded to the low price of some of the mutton brought to the Boston market. We do not wish the reader to infer that there is none other to be had: on the contrary, we have occasionally seen as good mutton there as in any European market. There are a number of practical and worthy men engaged in improving the different kinds of live stock, and preventing the degeneracy to which we refer. They have taken much interest in that class of stock, and they have been abundantly rewarded for their labor. But the great mass want more light on this subject, and for this reason we endeavor to show the causes of degeneracy, to enable them to avoid the errors of their forefathers.

Mr. Roberts, of Pennsylvania, says, " Early in my experience, I witnessed the renovation of a flock of what we call country sheep, that had been too long propagated in the same blood. This was about the year 1798. An imported ram from England, with heavy horns, very much resembling the most vigorous Spanish Merinoes, was obtained. The progeny were improved in the quality of fleece, and in the vigor of constitution. On running this stock in the same blood for some twelve years, a great deterioration became apparent. A male was then obtained of the large coarse-wooled Spanish stock: improvement in the vigor of the progeny was again most obvious. A Tunis mountain ram was then obtained, with a result equally favorable. In this process, fineness of fleece or weight was less the object than the carcass. In 1810, a male of not quite pure Merino blood was placed with the same stock of ewes; and a change of the male from year to year, for some time, produced a superior Merino stock Wool of a marketable quality for fine cloths was now the object; and it was not an unprofitable husbandry, when it would sell in the fleece, unwashed, from eighty-six cents to one dollar. The Saxon stock then became the rage, and the introduction of a tup of that country diminished greatly the weight of the fleece, without adequately improving its fineness. A male of the Spanish stock would give sometimes nine pounds; and the marsh graziers say that they went as high as fifteen pounds. Saxon males scarcely exceed five pounds, and the ewes two and a half pounds. By running in the same blood, and poor keeping, the fleece may be made finer, but it will be lightened in proportion, and of a weak and infirm texture. There are few stock-keepers who have mixed the Spanish with the Saxon breeds but what either do or will have cause to regret it. In this part of the country, a real Spanish Merino is not to be obtained. Sheep-raising has ceased to be a business of any profit nearer to the maritime coast than our extensive mountain ranges, whether for carcass or fleece. I sold, the last season, water-washed wool, of very fine quality, for thirty cents per pound. At such a price for wool, land near our seaports can be turned to better account, even in these dull times, than wool-growing. Stock sheep do best in stony and elevated locations, where they have to use diligence to pick the scanty blade. Sheep on the seaboard region should be kept more for carcass than fleece; and feeding, more than breeding, ought to be the object for some one hundred miles from tide water. It is now a well-ascertained fact, that health and vigor can only be perpetuated by not running too long on the same blood. The evils I have witnessed were due to a want of care on this head more than to any endemical quality in our climate. Sheep kept on smooth land and soft pasture are liable to the foot rot. The hoofs of the Merino require paring occasionally, for want of a stony mountain side to ascend. It is no longer a problem that this is to be a great wool-growing country, as well as a wool-consuming one. There is, in our wool-growing country and in abundance, held at a price that will enable the wool-grower to produce the finest qualities at thirty cents per pound, the cloths to be manufactured in proportion, and the market to be steady. I have seen Merino wool, since 1810, range from one dollar per pound to eighteen and three fourths cents, though I do not recollect selling below twenty-two cents. The best variety of sheep stock I have seen, putting fineness of fleece aside, was the mixed Bakewell and South Down, imported by Mr. Smith, of New Jersey. The flesh of the Merino has been pronounced of inferior flavor. This, however, does not agree with my experience, as I have found the lambs command a readier sale than any other, from being preferred by consumers."

DESCRIPTION OF THE DIFFERENT BREEDS OF SHEEP.

Mr. Lawson tells us that "the variety in sheep is so great, that scarcely any two countries produce sheep of the same kind. There is found a manifest difference in all, either in the size, the covering, the shape, or the horns.

TEESWATER BREED.

"This is a breed of sheep said to be the largest in England. It is at present the most prevalent in the rich, fine, fertile, enclosed lands on the banks of the Tees, in Yorkshire. In this breed, which is supposed to be from the same stock as those of the Lincolns, greater attention seems to have been paid to size than wool. It is, however, a breed only calculated for warm, rich pastures, where they are kept in small lots, in small enclosures, and well supported with food in severe winter seasons. The legs are longer, finer boned, and support a thicker and more firm and heavy carcass than the Lincolnshires; the sheep are much wider on the backs and sides, and afford a fatter and finer-grained mutton.

LINCOLNSHIRE BREED.

"This is a breed of sheep which is characterized by their having no horns; white faces; long, thin, weak carcasses; thick, rough, white legs; bones large; pelts thick; slow feeding; mutton coarse grained; the wool from ten to eighteen inches in length; and it is chiefly prevalent in the district which gives the name, and other rich grazing ones. The *new*, or improved Lincolns, have now finer bone, with broader loins and trussed carcasses, and are among the best, if not actually the best, long-wooled stock we have.

THE DISHLEY BREED.

"This is an improved breed of sheep, which is readily distinguished from the other long-wooled sorts; having a fulness of form and substantial width of carcass, with peculiar plainness and meekness of countenance; the head long, thin, and leaning backward; the nose projecting forward; the ears somewhat long, and standing backward; great fulness of the fore quarters; legs of moderate length, and the finest bone; tail small; fleece well covering the body, of the shortest and finest of the combing wools, the length of staple six or seven inches.

COTSWOLD BREED.

"This is a breed of sheep answering the following description: long, coarse head, with a particularly blunt, wide nose; a top-knot of wool on the forehead, running under the ears; rather long neck; great length and breadth of back and loin; full thigh, with more substance in the hinder than fore quarters; bone somewhat fine; legs not long; fleece soft, like that of the Dishley, but in closeness and darkness of color bearing more resemblance to short or carding wool. Although very fat, they have all the appearance of sheep that are full of solid flesh, which would come heavy to the scale. At two years and a half old, they have given from eleven to fourteen pounds of wool each sheep; and, being fat, they are indisputably among the larger breeds.

ROMNEY MARSH BREED.

"This is a kind which is described, by Mr. Young, as being a breed of sheep without horns; white faces and legs; rather long in the legs; good size; body rather long, but well barrel-shaped; bones rather large. In respect to the wool, it is fine, long, and of a delicate white color, when in its perfect state.

DEVONSHIRE BREED.

"This is a breed or sort of sheep which is chiefly distinguished by having no horns; white faces and legs; thick necks; backs narrow, and back-bones high; sides good; legs short, and bones large; and probably without any material objection, being a variety of the common hornless sort. Length of wool much the same as in the Romney Marsh breed. It is a breed found to be prevalent in the district from which it has derived its name, and is supposed to have received considerable improvement by being crossed with the new Leicester, or Dishley.

THE DORSETSHIRE BREED.

"This breed is known by having the face, nose, and legs white, head rather long, but broad, and the forehead woolly, as in the Spanish sort; the horn round and bold, middle-sized, and standing from the head; the shoulders broad at top, but lower than the hind quarters; the back tolerably straight; carcass deep, and loins broad; legs not long, nor very fine in the bone; the wool is fine and short. It is a breed which has the peculiar property of producing lambs at any period of the season, even so early as September and October, so as to suit the purposes of the lamb-suckler.

THE WILTSHIRE BREED.

"This is a sort which has sometimes the title of *horned crocks*. The writer on live stock distinguishes the breed as having a large head and eyes; Roman nose; wide nostrils; horns bending down the cheeks; color all white; wide bosom; deep, greyhound breast; back rather straight; carcass substantial; legs short; bone coarse; fine middle wool, very thin on the belly, which is sometimes bare. He supposes, with Culley, that the basis of this breed is doubtless the Dorsets, enlarged by some long-wooled cross; but how the horns came to take a direction so contrary, is not easy, he thinks, to conjecture; he has sometimes imagined it must be the result of some foreign, probably Tartarian cross.

THE SOUTH DOWN BREED.

"This is a valuable sort of sheep, which Culley has distinguished by having no horns; gray faces and legs; fine bones; long, small necks; and by being rather low before, high on the shoulder, and light in the fore quarter; sides good; loin tolerably broad; back-bone rather high; thigh full; twist good; mutton fine in grain and well flavored; wool short, very close and fine; in the length of the staple from two to three inches. It is a breed which prevails on the dry, chalky downs in Sussex, as well as the hills of Surrey and Kent, and which has lately been much improved, both in carcass and wool, being much enlarged forward, carrying a good fore flank; and for the short, less fertile, hilly pastures is an excellent sort, as feeding close. The sheep are hardy, and disposed to fatten quickly; and where the ewes are full kept, they frequently produce twin lambs, nearly in proportion of one third of the whole, which are, when dropped, well wooled.

THE HERDWICK BREED.

"This is a breed which is characterized by Mr. Culley as having no horns, and the face and legs being speckled; the larger portion of white, with fewer black spots, the purer the breed; legs fine, small, clean; the lambs well covered when dropped; the wool, short, thick, and matted in the fleece. It is a breed peculiar to the elevated, mountainous tract of country at the head of the River Esk, and Duddon in Cumberland, where they are let in herds, at an annual sum; whence the name. At present, they are said to possess the property of being extremely hardy in constitution, and capable of supporting themselves on the rocky, bare mountains, with the trifling support of a little hay in the winter season.

THE CHEVIOT BREED.

"This breed of sheep is known by the want of horns; by the face and legs being mostly white; little depth in the breast; narrow there and on the chine; clean, fine, small-boned legs, and thin pelts; the wool partly fine and partly coarse. It is a valuable breed of mountain sheep, where the herbage is chiefly of the natural grass kind, which is the case in the situations where these are found the most prevalent, and from which they have obtained their name. It is a breed which has undergone much improvement, within these few years, in respect to its form and other qualities, and has been lately introduced into the most northern districts; and from its hardiness, its affording a portion of fine wool, and being quick in fattening, it is likely to answer well in such situations.

THE MERINO BREED

'In this breed of sheep, the males have horns, but the females are without them. They have white faces and legs, the body not very perfect in shape ; rather long in the legs ; fine in the bone ; a production of loose, pendulous skin under the neck ; and the pelt fine and clear ; the wool very fine. It is a breed that is asserted by some to be tolerably hardy, and to possess a disposition to fatten readily.

THE WELSH SHEEP

"These, which are the most general breed in the hill districts, are small horned, and all over of a white color. They are neat, compact sheep. There is likewise a polled, short-wooled sort of sheep in these parts of the country, which are esteemed by some. The genuine Welsh mutton, from its smallness and delicate flavor, is commonly well known, highly esteemed, and sold at a high price."

SWINE.

PRELIMINARY REMARKS.

Swine have generally been considered "unclean," creatures of gross habits, &c.; but these epithets are unjust: they are not, in their nature, the unclean, gross, insensible brutes that mankind suppose them. If they are unclean, they got their first lessons from the lords of creation, by being confined in narrow, filthy sties — often deprived of light, and pure air, by being shut up in dark, underground cellars, to wallow in their own excrement; at other times, confined beneath stables, dragging out their existence in a perfect hotbed of corruption — respiring the emanations from the dung and urine of other animals; and often compelled to satisfy the cravings of hunger by partaking of whatever comes in their way. All manner of filth, including decaying and putrid vegetable and animal substances, are considered good enough for the hogs. And as long as they get such kind of trash, and no other, they must eat it; the cravings of hunger must be satisfied. The Almighty has endowed them with powerful organs of digestion; and as long as there is any thing before them that the gastric fluids are capable of assimilating, although it be disgusting to their very natures, rather than suffer of hunger, they will partake of it. Much of the indigestible food given to swine deranges the stomach, and destroys the powers of assimilation, or, in other words, leaves it in a morbid state. There is then a constant sensation of hunger, a longing for any and every thing within their reach. Does the reader wonder, then, at their morbid tastes? What will man do under the same circumstances? Suppose him to be the victim of dyspepsia or indigestion. In the early stages, he is constantly catering to the appetite. At one time, he longs for acids; at another, alkalies; now, he wants stimulants; then, refrigerants, &c. Again: what will not a man do to satisfy the cravings of hunger? Will he not eat his fellow, and drink of his blood? And all to satisfy the craving of an empty stomach.

We know from experience that, if young pigs are daily washed, and kept on clean cooked food, they will not eat the common city "swill;" they eat it only when compelled by hunger. When free from the control of man, they show as much sagacity in the selection of their food as any other animals; and, indeed, more than some, for they seldom get poisoned, like the ox, in mistaking noxious for wholesome food. The Jews, as well as our modern physiologists, consider the flesh of swine unfit for food. No doubt some of it is, especially that reared under the unfavorable circumstances alluded to above. But good home-fed pork, kept on good country produce, and not too fat, is just as good food for man as the flesh of oxen or sheep, notwithstanding the opinion of our medical brethren to the contrary. Their flesh has long been considered as one of the principal causes of scrofula, and other diseases too numerous to mention: without doubt this is the case. But that good, healthy pork should produce such results we are unwilling to admit. We force them to load their stomachs with the rotten offal of large cities, and thus derange their whole systems; they become loaded with fat; their systems abound in morbific fluids; their lungs become tuberculous; their livers enlarge; calcerous deposits or glandular disorganization sets in. Take into consideration their inactive habits; not voluntary, for instinct teaches them, when at liberty, to run, jump, and gambol, by which the excess of carbon is thrown off. Depriving them of exercise may be profitable to the breeder, but it induces a state of plethora. The cellular structures of such an animal are distended to their utmost capacity, preventing the full and free play of the vital machinery, obstructing the natural outlets (excrementitious vessels) on the external surface, and retaining in the system morbid materials that are positively injurious. At the present time, there is on exhibition in Boston a **woman,** styled the "fat girl;" she weighs four hundred and ninety-five pounds. A casual observer could detect nothing in her external appearance that denoted disease; yet she is liable to die at any moment from congestion of the brain, lungs, or liver. Any one possessing a knowledge of physiology would immediately pronounce her to be in a pathological state. Hence, the laws of the animal economy being uniform, we cannot arrive at any other conclusion in reference to the same plethoric state in animals of an inferior order.

Professor Liebig tells us that excess of carbon, in the form of food, cannot be employed to make a part of any organ; it must be deposited in the cellular tissue in the form of tallow or oil. This is the whole secret of fattening.

At every period of animal life, when there occurs a disproportion between the carbon of the food and the inspired oxygen, the latter being deficient, — which must happen beneath stables and in ill-constructed hog-sties, — fat must be formed.

Experience teaches us that in poultry the maximum of fat is obtained by preventing them from taking exercise, and by a medium temperature. These animals, in such circumstances, may be compared to a plant possessing in the highest degree the power of converting all food into parts of its own structure. The excess of the constituents of blood forms flesh and other organized tissues, while that of starch, sugar, &c., is converted into fat. When animals are fed on food destitute of nitrogen, only certain parts of their structure increase in size. Thus, in a goose fattened in the manner alluded to, the liver becomes three or four times larger than in the same animal when well fed, with free motion; while we cannot say that the organized structure of the liver is thereby increased. The liver of a goose fed in the ordinary way is firm and elastic; that of the imprisoned animal is soft and spongy. The difference consists in a greater or less expansion of its cells, which are filled with fat. Hence, when fat accumulates and free motion is prevented, the animal is in a diseased state. Now, many tons of pork are eaten in this diseased state, and it communicates disease to the human family: they blame the pork, when, in fact, the pork raisers are often more to blame. The reader is probably aware that some properties of food pass into the living organism without being assimilated by the digestive organs, and produce an abnormal state. For example, the faculty of New York have, time and again, testified to the destructive tendency of milk drawn from cows fed in cities, without due exercise and ordinary care in their management, giving it as their opinion that most of the diseases of children are brought about by its use. If proof were necessary to establish our position, we could cite it in abundance. A single case, which happened in our own family, will suffice. A liver, taken from an apparently healthy sow, (yet abounding in fat, and weighing about two hundred pounds,) was prepared in the usual manner for dinner. We observed, however, previous to its being cooked, that it was unusually large; yet there was no appearance of disease about it; it was quite firm. Each one partook of it freely. Towards night, and before partaking of any other kind of food, we were all seized with violent pains in the head, sickness at the stomach, and delirium: this continued for several hours, when a diarrhœa set in, through which process the offending matter was liberated, and each one rapidly recovered; pretty well convinced, however, that we had had a narrow escape, and that the liver was the sole cause of our misfortune.

Hence the proper management of swine becomes a subject of great importance; for, if more attention were paid to it, there would be less disease in the human family. When we charge these animals with being "unclean creatures of gross habits," let us consider whether we have not, in some measure, contributed to make them what they are.

Again: the hog has been termed "insensible," destitute of all those finer feelings that characterize brutes of a higher order. Yet we have "learned pigs," &c. — a proof that they can be taught something. A celebrated writer tells us that no animal has a greater sympathy for those of his own kind than the hog. The moment one of them gives a signal, all within hearing rush to his assistance. They have been known to gather round a dog that teased them and kill him on the spot; and if a male and female be enclosed in a sty when young, and be afterwards separated, the female will decline from the instant her companion is removed, and will probably die — perhaps of what would be termed, in the human family, a broken heart!

In the Island of Minorca, hogs are converted into beasts of draught; a cow, a sow, and two young horses, have been seen yoked together, and of the four the sow drew the best.

A gamekeeper of Sir H. Mildmay actually broke a sow to find game, and to back and stand.

Swine are frequently troubled with cutaneous diseases, which produce an itching sensation; hence their desire to wallow and roll in the mire and dirt. The lying down in wet, damp places relieves the irritation of the external surface, and cools their bodies. This mud and filth, however, in which they are often compelled to wallow, is by no means good or wholesome for them.

NATURAL HISTORY OF THE HOG.

"The hog," says Professor Low, "is subject to remarkable changes of form and characters, according to the situations in which he is placed. When these characters assume a certain degree of permanence, a breed or variety is formed; and there is none of the domestic animals which more easily receives the characters we desire to impress upon it. This arises from its rapid powers of increase, and the constancy with which the characters of the parents are reproduced in the progeny. *There is no kind of live stock that can be so easily improved by the breeder, and so quickly rendered suitable for the purposes required.*

"The body is large in proportion to the limbs, or, in other words, the limbs are short in proportion to the body; the extremities are free from coarseness; the chest is broad, and the trunk round. Possessing these characters, the hog neve fails to arrive at early maturity, and with a smaller consumption of food than when he possesses a different conformation.

"The wild boar, which was undoubtedly the progenitor of all the European varieties, and of the Chinese breed, was formerly a native of the British Islands, and very common in the forests until the time of the civil wars in that country."

We are told, that the wild hog "is now spread over the temperate and warmer parts of the old continent and its adjacent islands. His color varies with age and climate, but is generally a dusky brown, with black spots and streaks. His skin is covered with coarse hairs and bristles, intersected with soft wool, and with coarser and longer bristles upon the neck and spine, which he erects when in anger. He is a very bold and powerful creature, and becomes more fierce and indocile with age. From the form of his teeth, he is chiefly herbivorous in his habits, and delights in roots, which his acute sense of smell and touch enables him to discover beneath the surface. He also feeds on animal substances, such as worms and larvæ, which he grubs up from the earth, the eggs of birds, small reptiles, the young of animals, and occasionally carrion; he even attacks venomous snakes with impunity. In the natural state, the female produces a litter but once a year; * and

* In the domesticated state, the sow is often permitted to have two and even three litters in a year. This custom is very pernicious; it debilitates the mother, overworks all parts of the living machinery, and being in direct opposition to the laws of their being, their progeny must degenerate. Then, again, let the reader take into consideration the fact that members of the same litter impregnate each other, in the same ratio, and he cannot but

in much smaller numbers than when domesticated. She usually carries her young about four months.

"In the wild state, the hog has been known to live more than thirty years; but when domesticated, he is usually slaughtered before he is two years old. When the wild hog is tamed, it undergoes the following amongst other changes in its conformation: The ears become less movable, not being required to collect distant sounds; the formidable tusks of the male diminish, not being necessary for self-defence; the muscles of the neck become less developed, from not being so much exercised as in the natural state; the head becomes more inclined, the back and loins are lengthened, the body rendered more capacious, the limbs shorter and less muscular; and anatomy proves that the stomach and intestinal canals have also become proportionately extended along with the form of the body. The habits and instincts of the animal change; it becomes diurnal in its habits, not choosing the night for its search of food; is more insatiate in its appetite, and the tendency to obesity increases.

"The male, forsaking its solitary habits, becomes gregarious, and the female produces her young more frequently, and in larger numbers. With its diminished strength, and its want of active motion, the animal loses its desire for liberty.

"The true hog does not appear to be indigenous to America, but was taken over by the early voyagers from the old world, and it is now spread and multiplied throughout the continent.

"The first settlers of North America and the United States carried with them the swine of the parent country, and a few of the breeds still retain traces of the old English character. From its nature and habits, the hog was the most profitable and useful of all the animals bred by the early settlers in the distant clearings. It was his surest resource during the first years of toil and hardship."

Their widely-extended foreign commerce afforded the Amer-

come to a conclusion that we have long since arrived at — that these practices are among the chief causes of deterioration.

icans opportunity of procuring the varieties from China, Africa, and other countries. The large consumption of pork in the United States, and the facilities for disposing of it abroad, will probably cause more attention to be paid to the principles of breeding, rearing, feeding, &c. The American farmers are doing good service in this department, and any attempt on their part to improve the quality of pork ought to meet with a corresponding encouragement from the community. We have no doubt that many stock-raisers find their profits increase in proportion to the care bestowed in rearing. Here is an example: A Mr. Hallock, of the town of Coxsackie, has a sow which raised forty pigs within a year, which sold for $275, — none of them being kept over nine months. Mr. Little, of Poland, Ohio, states, in the Cultivator, that he has "a barrow three years old, a full-blood Berkshire, which will now weigh nearly 1000 pounds, live weight. He was weighed on the 3d of October, and then brought down 880; since which he has improved rapidly, and will doubtless reach the above figures. I have had this breed for seven years *pure*, — descended from hogs brought from Albany and Buffalo, and a boar imported by Mr. Fahnestock, of Pittsburg, Pa., from England, (the latter a very large animal.) The stock have all been large and very profitable — weighing, at seven to ten months old, from 250 to 300 pounds. Several individuals have weighed over 400, and the sire of this present one reached 750. This is, however, much the largest I have yet raised."

GENERALITIES.

Dr. Gunther observes, that "the robust constitution of the pig causes it to be less liable to fall sick than oxen and sheep. It would be still less liable to disease, if persons manifested more judgment in the choice of the animals to be reared, and if more care were shown in the matter. With reference to the latter point, it is very true that the voracity of the pig urges it to eat every thing it meets; but to keep it in a state of health, it is, notwithstanding, necessary to restrict its regimen to certain rules. The animal which it is proposed to fatten should remain under the roof, and receive good food there, whilst the others may be sent out for the greater part of the year, care being taken to avoid fields that are damp and marshy, and that the pigs be preserved from the dew. It is also of importance that they should not be driven too hard during warm days.

"There are two other points which deserve to be taken into consideration, if we wish swine to thrive: these are, daily exercise in the open air whenever the weather permits, and cleanliness in the sty. Constant confinement throws them into what may be called a morbid state, which renders their flesh less wholesome for man. The manner in which the animal evinces its joy when set at liberty proves sufficiently how disagreeable confinement is to it. A very general prejudice prevails, viz., that dung and filth do not injure swine; this opinion, however, is absurd."

GENERAL DEBILITY, OR EMACIATION.

THE falling off in flesh, or wasting away, of swine is in most cases owing to derangement in the digestive organs. The cure consists in restoring the tone of these organs. We commence the treatment by putting the animal on a boiled diet, consisting of bran, meal, or any wholesome vegetable production. The following tonic and diffusible stimulant will complete the cure: —

Powdered golden seal, . . .	}	equal parts.
" ginger, ...	}	

Dose a tea-spoonful, repeated night and morning.

When loss in condition is accompanied with cough and difficulty of breathing, mix, in addition to the above, a few kernels of garlic with the food. The drink should consist of pure water. Should the cough prove troublesome, take a tea-spoonful of fir balsam, and the same quantity of honey; to be given night and morning, either in the usual manner, or it may be stirred into the food while hot.

EPILEPSY, OR FITS.

The symptoms are too well known to need any description. It is generally caused by plethora, yet it may exist in an hereditary form.

Treatment. — Feed with due care, and put the animal in a well-ventilated and clean situation; give a bountiful supply of valerian tea, and sprinkle a small quantity of scraped horse-radish in the food; or give

Powdered assafœtida, ...	1 ounce.
" capsicum, ...	1 tea-spoonful.
Table salt, ...	1 table-spoonful.

Mix. Give half a tea-spoonful daily.

RHEUMATISM.

Causes. — Exposure, wallowing in filth, &c.

Symptoms. — It is recognized by a muscular rigidity of the whole system. The appetite is impaired, and the animal does not leave its sty willingly.

Treatment.—Keep the animal on a boiled diet, which should be given to him warm. Remove the cause by avoiding exposure and filth, and give a dose of the following:—

Powdered sulphur, ...		equal parts.
" sassafras, ...		
" cinnamon, ...		

Dose, half a tea-spoonful, to be given in warm gruel. If this does not give immediate relief, dip an old cloth in hot water, (of a proper temperature,) and fold it round the animal's body. This may be repeated, if necessary, until the muscular system is relaxed. The animal should be wiped dry, and placed in a warm situation, with a good bed of straw.

MEASLES.

This disease is very common, yet is often overlooked.

Symptoms.—It may be known by eruptions on the belly, ears, tongue, or eyelids. Before the eruption appears, the animal is drowsy, the eyes are dull, and there is sometimes loss of appetite, with vomiting. On the other hand, if the disease shall have receded towards the internal organs, its presence can only be determined by the general disturbance of the digestive organs, and the appearance of a few eruptions beneath the tongue.

Treatment.—Remove the animal from its companions to a warm place, and keep it on thin gruel. Give a tea-spoonful of sulphur daily, together with a drink of bittersweet tea. The object is to invite action to the surface, and maintain it there. If the eruption does not reappear on the surface, rub it with the following liniment:—

Take one ounce of oil of cedar; dissolve in a wine-glass

of alcohol; then add half a pint of new rum and a tea-spoonful of sulphur.

Almost all the diseases of the skin may be treated in the same manner.

OPHTHALMIA.

Causes. — Sudden changes in temperature, unclean sties, want of pure air, and imperfect light.

Treatment. — Keep the animal on thin gruel, and allow two tea-spoonfuls of cream of tartar per day. Wash the eyes with an infusion of marshmallows, until a cure is effected.

VERMIN.

Some animals are covered with vermin, which even pierce the skin, and sometimes come out by the mouth, nose, and eyes.

Symptoms. — The animal is continually rubbing and scratching itself, or burrowing in the dirt and mire.

Treatment. — First wash the body with a strong lie of wood ashes or weak saleratus water, then with an infusion of lobelia. Mix a tea-spoonful of sulphur, and the same quantity of powdered charcoal, in the food daily.

RED ERUPTION.

This disease is somewhat analogous to scarlet fever. It makes its appearance in the form of red pustules on the back and belly, which gradually extend to the whole body.

The external remedy is: —

Powdered bloodroot, ...	half an ounce.
Boiling vinegar, ...	1 pint.

When cool, it should be rubbed on the external surface.

The diet should consist of boiled vegetables, coarse meal, &c., with a small dose of sulphur every night.

DROPSY.

Symptoms. — The animal is sad and depressed, the appetite fails, respiration is performed with difficulty, and the belly swells.

Treatment. — Keep the animal on a light, nutritive diet, and give a handful of juniper berries, or cedar buds, daily. If these fail, give a table-spoonful of fir balsam daily.

CATARRH.

Symptoms. — Occasional fits of coughing, accompanied with a mucous discharge from the nose and mouth.

Causes. — Exposure to cold and damp weather.

Treatment. — Give a liberal allowance of gruel made with powdered elm or marshmallows, and give a tea-spoonful of balsam copaiba, or fir balsam, every night. The animal must be kept comfortably warm.

COLIC.

Spasmodic and flatulent colic requires antispasmodics and carminatives, in the following form: —

Powdered caraway seeds, .	1 tea-spoonful.
" assafœtida, . . .	one third of a tea-spoonful.

To be given at a dose in warm water, and repeated at the expiration of an hour, provided relief is not obtained.

DIARRHŒA.

For the treatment of this malady, see division Sheep, article *Scours*.

FRENZY.

This makes its appearance suddenly. The animal, having remained in a passive and stupid state, suddenly appears much disturbed, to such a degree that it makes irregular movements, strikes its head against every thing it meets, scrapes with its feet, places itself quite erect alongside of the sty, bites any thing in its way, and frequently whirls itself round, after which it suddenly becomes more tranquil.

Treatment. — Give half an ounce of Rochelle sa ts, in a pint of thoroughwort tea. If the bowels are not moved in the course of twelve hours, repeat the dose. A light diet for a few days will generally complete the cure.

JAUNDICE.

THIS disease is recognized by the yellow tint of the ***conjunctiva***, (white of the eye,) loss of appetite, &c.

The remedy is, —

Powdered golden seal,	. .	half an ounce.
" sulphur,	. . .	one fourth of an ounce.
" blue flag,	. . .	half an ounce.
Flaxseed,	. . . .	1 pound.

Mix, and divide into four parts, and give one every night. The food must be boiled, and a small quantity of salt added to it.

SORENESS OF THE FEET.

THIS often occurs to pigs that have travelled any distance: the feet often become tender and sore. In such cases, they should be examined, and all extraneous matter removed from the foot. Then wash with weak lie. If the feet discharge fetid matter, wash with the following mixture: —

Pyroligneous acid, ...	2 ounces.
Water, ...	4 ounces.

In the treatment of diseased swine, the "issues," as they are called, ought to be examined, and be kept free. They may be found on the inside of the legs, just above the pastern joint. They seem to serve as a drain or outlet for the morbid fluids of the body, and whenever they are obstructed, local or general disturbance is sure to supervene.

SPAYING.

THIS is the operation of removing the ovaries of sows, in order to prevent any future conception, and promote their fattening. (See article *Spaying Cows*, p. 201.) It is usually performed by making an incision in the middle of the flank, on the left side, in order to extirpate or cut off the ovaries, (female *testes*,) and then stitching up the wound, and wetting the part with Turlington's balsam. An able writer on this subject says, "The chief reason why a practice, which is beneficial in so many points of view to the interests and advantages of the farmer, has been so little attended to, is the difficulty which is constantly experienced from the want of a sufficient number of expert and proper persons to perform the operation. Such persons are far from being common in any, much less in every district, as some knowledge, of a nature which is not readily acquired, and much experience in the practice of cutting, are indispensably necessary to the success of the undertaking. When, however, the utility and benefits of the practice become better understood and more fully appreciated by the farmer, and the operators more numerous, much greater attention and importance will be bestowed upon it; as it is capable of relieving him from much trouble, of greatly promoting his profits, and of benefiting him in various ways. The facts are long since well proved and ascertained, that animals which have undergone this operation are more disposed to take on flesh, more quiet in their habits, and capable of being managed with much greater ease and facility in any way whatever, than they were before the operation was performed. It may also have advantages in other ways in different sorts of animals; it may render the filly nearly equal to the gelded colt for several different uses; and the heifer nearly equal to the ox for all sorts of farm labor. The females of some other sorts of animals may likewise, by this means, be made to nearly equal the castrated males in usefulness for a variety of purposes and intentions, and in all cases be rendered a good deal more valuable, or manageable, than they are at present."

VARIOUS BREEDS OF SWINE.

BERKSHIRE BREED.

This breed is distinguished by being in general of a tawny, white, or reddish color, spotted with black; large ears hanging over the eyes; thick, close, and well made in the body; legs short; small in the bone; having a disposition to fatten quickly. When well fed, the flesh is fine. The above county has long been celebrated for its breed of swine. The Berkshire breeders have made a very judicious use of the pug cross, by not repeating it to the degree of taking away all shape and power of growing flesh, in their stock. This breed is supposed by many to be the most hardy, both in respect to their nature and the food on which they are fed. Their powers of digestion are exceedingly energetic, and they require constant good keep, or they will lose flesh very fast. They thrive well in the United States, provided, however, due care is exercised in breeding.

HAMPSHIRE BREED.

This breed is distinguished by being longer in the body and neck, but not of so compact a form as the Berkshire. They are mostly of a white color, or spotted, and are easily fattened. The goodness of the Hampshire hog is proverbial and in England they are generally fattened for hams.

SHROPSHIRE BREED.

These are not so well formed as those of the Berkshire kind, or equal to them in their disposition to fatten, or to be supported on such cheap food. Their color is white or brinded. They are flat boned; deep and flat sided; harsh, or rather wiry-haired; the ear large; head long, sharp, and coarse; legs long; loin, although very substantial, yet not sufficiently wide, considering the great extent of the whole frame. They have been much improved by the Berkshire cross.

There are various other breeds, which take their name from the different counties in the mother country. Thus we have the Herefordshire, Wiltshire, Yorkshire, &c. Yet they are not considered equal to those already alluded to. Many of the different English breeds might, however, serve to im prove some species of breed in this country.

CHINESE BREED.

This is of small size; the body being very close, compact, and well formed; the legs very short; the flesh delicate and firm. The prevailing color, in China, is white. They fatten very expeditiously on a small quantity of food, and might be reared in the United States to good advantage, especially for home consumption.

BOARS AND SOWS FOR BREEDING.

Mr. Lawson says, "The best stock may be expected from the boar at his full growth, but no more than from three to five years old.* No sows should be kept open for breeding unless they have large, capacious bellies.

"It may be remarked, in respect to the period of being with young, that in the sow it is about four months; and the usual produce is about eight to ten or twelve pigs in the large, but more in the smaller breeds.

"In the ordinary management of swine, sows, after they have had a few litters, may be killed; but no breeder should part with one while she continues to bring good litters, and rear them with safety."

Pregnant sows should always be lodged separately, especially at the time of bringing forth their young, else the pigs would most probably be devoured as they fall. The sow should also be attended with due care while pigging, in order to preserve the pigs. It is found that dry, warm, comfortable lodging is of almost as much importance as food. The pigs may be weaned in about eight weeks, after which the sow requires less food than she does while nursing. In the management of these animals, it is of great utility and advantage to separate the males from the females, as it lessens their sexual desires.

REARING PIGS.

"As the breeding of pigs is a business that affords the farmer a considerable profit and advantage in various views, it is of essential importance that he be provided with suitable kinds of food in abundance for their support. Upon this being properly and effectually done, his success and advantage will in a great measure depend. The crops capable of being cultivated with the most benefit in this intention are, beans,

* Sows are generally bred from too early—before they come to maturity. This not only stints their own growth, but their offspring give evidence of deterioration. A sow should never be put to the boar until she be a year old.

peas, barley, buckwheat, Indian corn, potatoes, carrots, parsnips, Swedish turnips, cabbages, &c.

"The sows considerably advanced in pig, and those with pigs, should be fed in a better manner than the stone pigs. The former should be supplied with boiled meal, potatoes, carrots, &c., so as to keep them in good condition. The sows with pigs should be kept with the litters in separate sties, and be still better fed than those with pig. When dairying is practised, the wash of that kind which has been preserved for that purpose while the dairying was profitable, must be given them, with food of the root kind, such as carrots, parsnips, &c., in as large proportions as they will need to keep them in condition."

Pea-soup is an admirable article when given in this intention; it is prepared by boiling six pecks of peas in about sixty gallons of water, till they are well broken down and diffused in the fluid: it is then put into a tub or cistern for use. When dry food is given in combination with this, or of itself, the above writer advises oats, as being much better than any other sort of grain for young pigs, barley not answering nearly so well in this application. Oats coarsely ground have been found very useful for young hogs, both in the form of wash with water, and when made of a somewhat thicker consistence. But in cases where the sows and pigs can be supported with dairy-wash and roots, as above, there will be a considerable saving made, by avoiding the use of the expensive articles of barley-meal, peas, or bran.

Mr. Donaldson remarks, that in the usual mode, the pigs reared by the farmer are fed, for some weeks after they are weaned, on whey or buttermilk, or on bran or barley-meal mixed with water. They are afterwards maintained on other food, as potatoes, carrots, the refuse of the garden, kitchen, scullery, &c., together with such additions as they can pick up in the farm-yard. Sometimes they are sent into the fields at the close of harvest, where they make a comfortable living for several weeks on the gleanings of the crop; at other times, when the farm is situated in the neighborhood of woods or forests, they are sent thither to pick up the beech-nuts and acorns in the fall of the year; and when they have arrived at a proper age for fattening, they are either put into sties fitted up for the purpose, or sold to distillers, starch-makers, dairymen, or cottagers.

Nothing tends more effectually to preserve the health and promote the growth of young pigs than the liberal use of hay tea. The tea should be thickened with corn meal and shorts. This, given lukewarm, twice a day, will quicken their growth, and give the meat a rich flavor. A few parsnips * or carrots (boiled) may be made use of with much success.

FATTENING HOGS.

F. Dodge, of Danvers, Mass., states that, in the spring of 1848, he "bought, from a drove, seven shotes, the total weight of which was 925 pounds. The price paid for them was seven cents per pound. They were fed an average of 184 days, and their average gain was 179 pounds of net pork. The cost of the food they consumed was as follows: —

68 bushels corn at 53 cents,	$36 04
30 " " damaged, at 35 cents	10 50
50 " " at 65 cents,	32 50
8 " meal at 65 cents,	5 20
	$84 24
Add first cost of pigs,	64 75
Making a total cost of	$148 99

"The whole quantity of pork afforded by the pigs killed was 2178 pounds, which was sold at 6½ cents per pound, amounting

* The Sussex (Eng.) Express says, "At our farm we have been in the habit of employing parsnips for this purpose for some time. Upon reference to our books, we find that on the 11th of October, 1847, we put up two shotes of eleven weeks old, and fed them on skim milk and parsnips for three months, when they were killed, weighing 231 and 238 pounds. They were well fattened, firm in flesh, and the meat of excellent flavor. The quantity of parsnips consumed by them was nine bushels each."

to $141 57; leaving a balance against the pigs of $7 42. The inference from this statement is, that, at the above prices of grain, pork could not be profitably produced at six and a half cents per pound. But it is suggested that something might be saved by breeding the stock, instead of purchasing shotes at seven cents per pound, live weight. It is thought, however, that the manure afforded by the hogs would be of sufficient value to more than overbalance any deficiency which might appear in the account by only crediting the pork."

The food in the above case was too costly. One half of it, mixed with parsnips, carrots, beets, or turnips, would have answered the purpose better. The balance would then have been in favor of the pigs. We are told, by an able writer on swine, that they will feed greedily, and thrive surprisingly, on most kinds of roots and tubers, such as carrots, beets, parsnips, potatoes, &c., particularly when prepared by boiling. It may be taken as a general rule, that boiled or prepared food is more nutritious and fattening than raw or cold food; the additional expense and labor will be more than compensated by the increased weight and quality.

Cornstalks might be used as food for swine by first cutting them * in small pieces, and then boiling them until they are quite soft; a small quantity of meal is then to be mixed in the fluid, and the stalks again added, and fed to the pigs twice a day.

Mr. P. Wing, of Farmersville, C. W., gives us his experience in feeding swine; and he requests his brother farmers to make similar experiments with various kinds of food, and, by preparing them in various ways, to ascertain what way it will yield the most nutriment — that is, make the most pork. He says, —

"I now give the result of feeding 100 bushels of good peas to sixteen hogs, of various mixed breeds, as found in this section. The peas were boiled until fine, making what I call thick soup. After having fed the hogs on the same kind

* Messrs. Parker & White, in Boston, have shown us an excellent machine used for the purpose of cutting cornstalks. Every farmer should have one in his possession.

of food for two weeks, I gave them their morning feed, and weighed each one separately, noting the weight. Twelve of them were about eighteen months old; one was a three year old sow, and three pigs were seven and a half months old when weighed. I found their total weight 4267 lbs.; and after consuming the above amount, which took forty-two days, I weighed them again, and found that they had gained 1358 lbs.; and on the supposition that as they gained in flesh they shrunk in offal, I estimated their net gain to have been 1400 lbs. Their drink consisted of ten pails of whey per day. It was allowed to stand forty-eight hours, and the cream was skimmed off.

"I find that there is a great difference in breeds of hogs. The three year old sow was small framed, and pretty full-fleshed, weighing 504 lbs. Her gain in the forty-two days was 66 lbs. The three pigs were from her, and showed traces of three distinct breeds of hogs. Their first weight and gain were as follows: the first weighed 253 lbs. — gain, 97 lbs.; the second, 218 lbs. — gain, 75 lbs.; the third, 171 lbs. — gain, 46 lbs. When butchered, the smallest one was the best pork, being the fattest. Two of the most inferior of the hogs gained 1½ lbs. per day; six, a mixture of the Berkshire, (I should think about one fourth,) gained 1¾ lbs. per day; three of the common stock of our country gained 2½ lbs.; and one of a superior kind weighed 318 lbs., and in the forty-two days gained 134 lbs. They were weighed on the 20th September, the first time. They were kept confined in a close pen, except once a week I let them out for exercise, and to wallow, for the most part of a day."

METHOD OF CURING SWINE'S FLESH.

"In the county of Kent, when pork is to be cured as bacon, it is the practice to singe off the hairs by making a straw fire round the carcass — an operation which is termed *swaling.* The skin, in this process, should be kept perfectly free from dirt of all sorts. When the flitches are cut out, they should be rubbed effectually with a mixture of common salt and saltpetre, and afterwards laid in a trough, where they are to continue three weeks or a month, according to their size, keeping them frequently turned; and then, being taken out of the trough, are to be dried by a slack fire, which will take up an equal portion of time with the former; after which, they are to be hung up, or thrown upon a rack, there to remain until wanted. But in curing bacon on the continent, it is mostly the custom to have closets contrived in the chimneys, for the purpose of drying and smoking by wood fires, which is said to be more proper for the purpose. And a more usual mode of curing this sort of meat is that of salting it down for pickled pork, which is far more profitable than bacon.

"In the county of Westmoreland, where the curing of hams has long been practised with much success, the usual method is for them to be at first rubbed very hard with bay salt; by some they are covered close up; by others they are left on a stone bench, to allow the brine and blood to run off. At the end of five days, they are again rubbed, as hard as they were at first, with salt of the same sort, mixed with an ounce of saltpetre to a ham. Having lain about a week, either on a stone bench or in hogsheads amongst the brine, they are hung up, by some in the chimney, amidst the smoke, whether of peat or coals; by others in places where the smoke never reaches them. If not sold sooner, they are suffered to remain there till the weather becomes warm. They are then packed in hogsheads with straw or oatmeal husks, and sent to the place of sale."

A small portion of pyroligneous acid may be added to the brine. It is a good antiseptic, and improves the flavor of ham and bacon. (See *Acid, Pyroligneous*, in the *Materia Medica.*)

APPENDIX.

ON THE ACTION OF MEDICINES.

In reference to the action of medicines and external agents on the animal body, we would observe, that warmth and moisture always expand it, and bayberry bark, tannin, and gum catechu always contract it; and that these agents have these effects at all times (provided, however, there be sufficient vitality in the part to manifest these peculiar changes) and under all circumstances. If a blister be applied to the external surface of an animal, and it produces irritation, it always has a tendency to produce that effect, whatever part of the living organism it may be applied to. So alcohol always has a tendency to stimulate; whether given by the mouth, or rubbed on the external surface, it will produce an excitement of nerves, heart, and arteries, and of course the muscles partake of the influence. Again, marshmallows, gum acacia, slippery elm, &c., always lubricate the mucous surfaces, quiet irritation, and relieve inflammatory symptoms.

It follows, of course, 1st. That when any other effects than those just named are seen to follow the administration of these articles, they must be attributed to the morbid state of the parts to which they are applied; 2d. That a medicine which is good to promote a given effect in one form of disease, will be equally good for the same purpose in another form of disease in the same tissue. Thus, if an infusion of mallows is good for inflammation of the stomach, and will lubricate the surface, and allay irritation in that organ, then it is equally good for the same purpose in inflammation of the bowels and bladder. What we wish the reader to understand is this: that a medicine used for any particular symptom in one form of disease, if it be a sanative agent, is equally good for the same symptom in every form. Medical men range their various remedies under different heads. Thus opium is called narcotic, aloes purgative or cathartic, potass diuretic, &c. And because the same results do not always follow the administration of these articles, they are perplexed, and are compelled to try every new remedy, in hopes to find a specific; not knowing that many of their "*best medicines*" (opium, for example) war against the vital principle, and as soon as they get into the system, nature sets up a strong action to counteract their effects; in short, to get them out of the system in the quickest possible manner: sometimes they pass through the kidneys; at other times, the intestinal canal, the lungs, or surface, afford them egress. And because a certain agent does not always act in their hands with unerring certainty, they seem to suppose that the same uncertainty attends the administration of every article in the *materia medica.* The medicines we recommend owe their diuretic, astringent, diaphoretic, and cathartic powers to their aromatic, relaxing, antispasmodic, lubricating, and irritating properties; and if we give them with a view of producing a certain result, and they do not act just as we wish, it is no proof that they have not done good. The fact is, all our medicines act on the parts where nature is making the greatest efforts to restore equilibrium; hence they relieve the constitution, whatever may be the nature of their results.

Many of the remedies recommended in this work are denounced by the United States Dispensatory as "useless, inert," &c.; yet many of our most celebrated physicians are in the daily habit of using them. Mr. Bracy Clark, V. S., recommends tincture of allspice for gripes. And Mr. Causer, an experienced veterinarian, says, "I ordered a dessert spoonful (about two drachms) of tincture of gentian and bark to be given twice a day in a case of gripes. Scarcely an hour after the animal had taken the first dose, he began to eat some hay, and on the next day he ate every thing that was offered him. After this, I ordered a quart of cold boiled milk to be given him every morning and evening. By these means, together with the good care of the coachman, he recovered his strength." Mr. White, V. S., says, "I have been assured by a veterinary surgeon, that he once cured a horse of gripes by a dose of hot water; and it is by no means unlikely that a warm infusion of some of our medicinal herbs, such as peppermint, pennyroyal, rosemary, &c., would be found effectual."

Mr. Gibson says, "It is a fact that cannot be too generally known, that an infusion of garlic has, to my certain knowledge, cured several cases of epilepsy — a dreadful disease, that seems to have baffled, in most instances, every effort of medical skill."

An intelligent farmer assures Dr. White that he has had forty sheep at a time hoven or blasted from feeding on vetches, and so swollen that he hardly knew which would drop first. His usual remedy was a quart of water for each sheep; and that generally had the desired effect, though many died before it could be given. We might give our own experience in favor of numberless simple agents, which we are in the constant habit of using, were it necessary; suffice it to say, that at the present time we use nothing else than simple means.

CLYSTERS.

Remarks. — As the more general use of clysters is recommended by the author, especially in acute diseases, he has thought proper to introduce, in this part of the work, a few remarks on them, with examples of their different forms. They serve not only to evacuate the rectum of its contents.

but assist to evacuate the intestines, and serve also to convey nourishment into the system; as in cases of locked-jaw, and great prostration. They soften the hardened excrement in the rectum, and cause it to be expelled · besides, by their warm and relaxing powers, they act as fomentations. A stimulating clyster in congestion of the brain, or lungs, will relieve those parts by counter-irritation. An animal that is unable to swallow may be supported by nourishing clysters; for the lacteals, which open into the inner cavity of the intestines, absorb, or take up, the nourishment, and convey it into the thoracic duct, as already described. Some persons deny the utility of injections. We are satisfied on that point, and are able to convince any one, beyond a reasonable doubt, that fluids are absorbed in the rectum, notwithstanding the opinion of some men to the contrary.

In administering clysters, it ought always to be observed that the fluids should be neither too hot nor too cold: they should be about the temperature of the blood. The common sixteen-ounce metal syringe, with a wooden pipe about six inches in length, and gradually tapering from base to point, is to be preferred. It is, after being oiled, much more easily introduced into the fundament than one that is considerably smaller; and, having a blunt point, there is no danger of hurting the animal, or wounding the rectum.

The following injections are suitable for all kinds of animals. The quantity, however, should be regulated according to the size of the patient. Thus a quart will suffice for a sheep or pig, while three or four quarts are generally necessary in the case of horses and cattle. If clysters are intended to have a nutritive effect, they must be introduced in the most gentle manner, and not more than one pint should be given at any one time, for fear of exciting the expulsive action of the rectum. In constriction and intussusception of the intestines, and when relaxing clysters are indicated, they should not be too long persevered in, for falling of the rectum has been known, in many instances, to arise from repeated injections. Efforts should be made to relax the whole animal by warmth and moisture externally, and in the use of antispasmodic teas rather than to place too much dependence on clysters.

FORMS OF CLYSTERS.

Laxative Clyster.

Warm water, ...	3 or 4 quarts.
Linseed oil, ...	8 ounces.
Common salt, (fine,)	1 table-spoonful.

Another.

Warm water, ...	4 quarts.
Soft soap, ...	1 gill.
Fine salt, ...	half a table-spoonful.

Use. — Either of the above clysters is useful in obstinate constipation, "stoppage," or whenever the excrement is hard and dark colored.

Emollient Clyster.

Slippery elm bark, ...	2 ounces.
Boiling water, ...	2 quarts.

Let them simmer over the fire for a few minutes, then strain through a fine sieve, and inject. The following articles may be substituted for elm: flaxseed, lily roots, gum arabic, poplar bark, Iceland moss.

Use. — In all cases of irritation and inflammation of the intestines and bladder.

Stimulating Clyster.

Thin mucilage of slippery elm or linseed tea, ...	3 quarts.
African cayenne *	1 tea-spoonful.

* A large portion of the cayenne found in the stores is adulterated with logwood, and is positively injurious, as it would thus prove astringent

Another

Powdered ginger, ...	half a table-spoonful.
Boiling water, ...	3 quarts.

When cool, inject.

Use. — In all cases, when the rectum and small intestines are inactive, and loaded with excrement, or gas.

Anodyne Clyster.

Lady's slipper, (*cypripedium,*) . . .	1 ounce.
Camomile flowers, ...	1 ounce.
Boiling water, ...	3 quarts.

Let the mixture stand a short time, then strain through a fine sieve, when it will be fit for use.

Use. — To relieve pain and relax spasms.

Diuretic Clyster.

Linseed tea, ...	3 quarts.
Oil of juniper, ...	1 table-spoonful.

Or, substitute for the latter, cream of tartar, half an ounce.

Use. — This form of clyster may be used with decided advantage in all acute diseases of the urinary organs. This injection is useful in cases of red water, both in cattle and sheep; and when the malady is supposed to result from general or local debility, the addition of tonics (golden seal or gentian *) will be indicated.

Astringent Clyster.

Take an infusion of hardhack, strain, and add a table-spoonful of finely-pulverized charcoal to every three quarts of fluid.

* Their active properties may be extracted by infusion.

Another.

An infusion of witch hazel.

Another.

Powdered bayberry bark, . . .	1 table-spoonful.
Boiling water, ...	3 quarts

When cool, it is fit for use.

Use. — Astringent injections are used in all cases where it is desired to contract the living fibre, as in scouring, dysentery, scouring rot, diarrhœa, bloody flux, falling of the womb, fundament, &c.

Nourishing Clyster.

Nourishing clysters are composed of thin gruel made from flour, &c.

Injection for Worms.

Make an infusion of pomegranate, (rind of the fruit,) and inject every night for a few days. This will rid the animal of worms that infest the rectum; but if the animal is infested with the long, round worm, (*teres*,) then half a pint of the above infusion must be given for a few mornings, before feeding.

Another for Worms.

Powdered lobelia, ...	1 ounce.
Wood ashes, ...	a handful.
Boiling water, ...	3 quarts.

When cool, it is fit for use.

INFUSIONS.

These are made by steeping herbs, roots, and other medicinal substances in boiling water. No particular rules can be laid down as to the quantity of each article required: it will, however, serve as some sort of a guide, to inform the reader that we generally use from one to two ounces of the aromatic herbs and roots to every quart of fluid. A bitter infusion, such as wormwood or camomile, requires less of the herb. All kinds of infusions can be rendered palatable by the addition of a small quantity of honey or molasses. As a general rule, the human palate is a good criterion; for if an infusion be too strong or unpalatable for man, it is unfit for cattle or sheep. We do not depend so much on the strength of our agents: the great secret is to select the one best adapted to the case in view. If it be an agent that is capable of acting in concert with nature, then the weaker it is, the better. In short, nature requires but slight assistance under all ordinary circumstances, unless the animal is evidently suffering from debility; then our efforts must act in concert with the living powers. We must select the most nutritious food—that which can be easily converted into blood, bones, and muscles. If, on the other hand, we gave an abundance of provender, and it lacked the constituents necessary for the purposes in view, or was of such an indigestible nature that its nutritive properties could not be extracted by the gastric fluids, this would be just as bad as giving improper medicines, both in reference to its quantity and quality.

An infusion of either of the following articles is valuable in colic, both flatulent and spasmodic, in all classes of animals: caraways, peppermint, spearmint, fennel-seed, angelica, bergamot, snakeroot, aniseed, ginseng, &c.

ANTISPASMODICS.

By antispasmodics are meant those articles that assist, through their physiological action, in relaxing the nervous and muscular systems. Hence the reader will perceive, by the definition we have given of this class of remedies, that we cannot recommend or employ the agents used by our brethren of the allopathic school, for many of them act pathologically. The class we use are simple, yet none the the less efficient.

Professor Curtis says, when alluding to the action of medicinal agents, "Experiments have shown that many vegetable substances, which seem in themselves quite bland and harmless, are antidotes to various poisons. Thus the skull-cap (*scutellaria laterifolia*) is said to be a remedy for hydrophobia, the *alisma plantago* and *polemonium reptans* for the bites of serpents, and lobelia for the sting of insects. They are good; but why? Because they are permanently relaxing and stimulating, and depurate the whole system."

Natural antispasmodics are warmth and moisture. The medicinal ones are lobelia, Indian hemp, castor musk, ginseng assafœtida, pleurisy root, Virginia snakeroot, camomile, wormwood. The above are only specimens. There is no limit to the number and variety of articles in the vegetable kingdom that will act as antispasmodics or relaxants. They may be given internally or applied externally: the effect is the same.

FOMENTATIONS.

This class of remedies is usually composed of relaxants, &c., of several kinds, combined with tonics, stimulants, and anodynes. They are very useful to relieve pain, to remove rigidity, to restore tone, and to stimulate the parts to which they are applied.

Common Fomentation.

Wormwood,	. . . .	equal parts.
Tansy,	. . . .	
Hops,	. . . .	

Moisten them with equal parts of boiling water and vinegar, and apply them blood warm.

Use.—For all kinds of bruises and sprains. They should be confined to the injured parts, and kept moist with the superabundant fluid. When it is not practicable to confine a fomentation to the injured parts, as in shoulder or hip lameness, constant bathing with the decoction will answer the same purpose.

Anodyne Fomentation.

Hops, ...	a handful.
White poppy heads, ...	1 ounce.
Water and vinegar, ...	equal parts.

Simmer a few minutes.

Use.—In all painful bruises.

Relaxing Fomentation.

Powdered lobelia, ...	2 ounces.
Boiling water, ...	2 quarts.

Simmer for a few minutes, and when sufficiently cool, bathe the parts with a soft sponge.

Use.—In all cases of stiff joints, and rigidity of the muscles. Animals often lie down in wet pastures, from which rheumatism and stiffness of the joints arise. In such cases, the animal must be taken from grass for a few days, and the affected parts be faithfully bathed.

Stimulating Fomentation.

Cedar buds, or boughs, any quantity, to which add a

small quantity of red pepper and ginger, boiling water sufficient.

Use. — This will be found very efficacious in chronic lameness and paralysis, for putrid sore throat, and when the gland are enlarged from cold and catarrh.

MUCILAGES.

Mucilages are soft, bland substances, made by dissolving gum arabic in hot water; or by boiling marshmallows, slippery elm, or lily roots, until their mucilaginous properties are extracted. A table-spoonful of either of the above articles, when powdered, will generally suffice for a quart of water.

Use. — In all cases of catarrh, diarrhœa, inflammation of the kidneys, womb, bladder, and intestines. They shield the mucous membranes, and defend them from the action of poisons and drastic cathartics.

WASHES.

Washes generally contain some medicinal agent, and are principally used externally.

Wash for Diseases of the Feet.

Pyroligneous acid, ...	4 ounces.
Water, ...	8 ounces.

Use. — This wash excels every other in point of efficacy, and removes rot and its kindred diseases sooner than any other.

Cooling Wash for the Eye.

Rain water, ...	1 pint.
Acetic acid, ...	20 drops.

Use. — In ophthalmia.

Tonic and Antispasmodic Wash.

Camomile flowers, ...	half an ounce.
Boiling water, ...	1 pint.

When cool, strain through fine linen.

Use. —In chronic diseases of the eye, and when a weeping remains after an acute attack.

Wash for unhealthy (or ulcerated) Sores.

A weak solution of sal soda or wood ashes.

Wash for Diseases of the Skin.

Take one ounce of finely-pulverized charcoal, pour on it one ounce of pyroligneous acid, then add a pint of water. Bottle, and keep it well corked. It may be applied to the skin by means of a sponge. It is also an excellent remedy for ill-conditioned ulcers.

PHYSIC FOR CATTLE.

Extract of butternut, (*juglans cinerea,*) .	half an ounce.
Cream of tartar, ...	1 tea-spoonful.
Boiling water, ...	2 quarts.

Mix. When cool, administer.

Another.

Extract of blackroot, (*leptandra virginica*,) .	half an ounce.
Rochelle salts, ...	1 ounce.
Powdered ginger, ...	½ tea-spoonful.

Dissolve in two quarts of warm water.

Another.

Powdered mandrake, ...	1 table-spoonful.
Cream of tartar, ...	1 tea-spoonful.
Hot water	2 quarts.

Here are three different forms of physic for cattle, which do not debilitate the system, like aloes and salts, because they determine to the surface as well as the bowels. They may be given in all cases where purges are necessary. One third of the above forms will suffice for sheep.

MILD PHYSIC FOR CATTLE.

Sirup of buckthorn, ...	2 ounces.
Sulphur, ...	half a table-spoonful
Ginger, ...	half a tea-spoonful.
Hot water, ...	2 quarts.

Aperient.

Linseed oil, ...	1 pint.
Yolks of two eggs.	

Mix.

Another.

Sweet oil, ...	1 pint.
Powdered cayenne, ...	half a tea-spoonful.

Mix.

A sheep will require about one half of the above.

Stimulating Tincture.

Boiling vinegar, ...	1 pint.
Tincture of myrrh, ...	2 ounces.
Powdered capsicum, ...	2 tea-spoonfuls.

Use. — For external application in putrid sore throat.

Another.

Tincture of camphor, ...	4 ounces.
Oil of cedar, ...	half an ounce.
Tincture of capsicum, (hot drops,) .	4 ounces.

To be rubbed around the throat night and morning.

Stimulating Tincture for Chronic Rheumatism.

Tincture of capsicum, ...	4 ounces.
Oil of cedar, ...	1 ounce.
Oil of wormwood, ...	1 ounce.
Vinegar, ...	half a pint.
Goose grease, ...	1 gill.

Mix. To be applied night and morning. The mixture should be kept in a well-corked bottle, and shaken before being used.

POULTICES.

Preliminary Remarks. — As oxen, sheep, and pigs are liable to have accumulations of matter, in the form of abscess, resulting from injury or from the natural termination of diseases, it becomes a matter of importance that the farmer should rightly understand their character and treatment. If a foreign substance enters the flesh, the formation of matter is a part of the process by which nature rids the system of the enemy. A poultice relaxing and lubricating will then be indicated. If, however, the foreign body shall have entered at a point where it is impossible to confine a poultice, then the suppurative stage may be shortened by the application of relaxing fomentations, and lastly, by stimulants. It is a law of the animal economy, that, unless there be some obstacle, matter always seeks its exit by an external opening; and it becomes part of our duty to aid nature in her efforts to accomplish this salutary object. Nature requires aid in consequence of the unyielding character of the hide, and the length of time it takes to effect an opening through it. Animals are known to suffer immensely from the pressure a large accumulation of pus makes on the surrounding nerves, &c., and also from the reabsorption of this pus when it cannot readily make its exit. This is not all; for, if pus accumulates, and cannot in due time find an outlet, it produces destruction of the blood-vessels, nerves, and surrounding tissues. These vessels are distributed to the different surfaces; their supply of blood and nervous energy being cut off, they decompose, and in their turn become pus, and their open mouths allow the morbid matter to enter the circulation, and thus poison the blood. Hence it becomes our duty, whenever matter can be distinctly felt, to apply that sort of poultice which will be most likely to aid nature.

There is no article in the *materia medica* of so much value to the farmer as marshmallows; he cannot place too much value on it. Whether he uses it in his own family or confines it exclusively to cattle practice, it is equally valuable. It has numerous advantages over many similar remedies: the most important one to the farmer is, that it can be procured in this country at a small cost. We have used it for a number of years, and in many cases we consider it our sheet-anchor. In short, we cannot supply its place.

Mr. Cobbett says, "I cannot help mentioning another herb, which is used for medicinal purposes. I mean the marshmallows. It is amongst the most valuable of plants that ever grew Its leaves stewed, and applied wet, will cure, and almost instantly cure, any cut, or bruise, or wound of any sort. Poultices made of it will cure sprains; fomenting with it will remove swellings; applications of the liquor will cure chafes made by saddles and harness; and its operation, in all cases, is so quick that it is hardly to be believed. Those who have this weed at hand need not put themselves to the trouble and expense of sending to doctors and farriers on trifling occasions. It signifies not whether the wound be old or new. The mallows, if you have it growing near you, may be used directly after it is gathered, merely washing off the dirt first. But there should be some always ready in the house for use. It should be gathered just before it blooms, and dried and preserved just in the same manner as other herbs. It should be observed, however, that, if it should happen not to be gathered at the best season, it may be gathered at any time. I had two striking instances of the efficacy of mallows. A neighboring farmer had cut his thumb in a very dangerous manner, and, after a great deal of *doctoring*, it had got to such a pitch that his hand was swelled to twice its natural size. I recommended the use of the mallows to him, gave him a little bunch out of my store, (it being winter time,) and his hand was well in four days. He could go out to his work the very next day, after having applied the mallows over night. The other instance was this. I had a valuable hog, that had been gored by a cow. It had been in this state for two days before I knew of the accident, and had eaten nothing. The gore was in the side, making a large wound. I poured in the liquor in which the mallows had been stewed, and rubbed the side well with it. The next day the hog got up and began to eat. On examining the wound, I found it so far closed that I did not think it right to disturb it. I bathed the side again; and in two days the hog was turned out, and was running about along with the rest. Now, a person must be criminally careless not to make provision of this herb. Mine was nearly two years old when I made use of it upon the last-mentioned occasion. If the use of this weed was generally adopted the art and mystery of healing wounds, and of curing sprains, swellings, and other external maladies, would very quickly be reduced to an unprofitable trade."

Lubricating and healing Poultice.

Powdered marshmallow roots, . .	equal parts.
Marshmallow leaves, ...	

Moisten with boiling water, and apply.

Use. — In ragged cuts, wounds, and bruises.

Stimulating Poultice.

Indian meal, ...	equal parts.
Slippery elm, ...	

Mix them together, and add sufficient boiling water to moisten the mass. Spread it on a cloth, and sprinkle a small quantity of powdered cayenne on its surface.

Use. — To stimulate ill-conditioned ulcers to healthy action. Where there is danger of putrescence, add a small quantity of powdered charcoal.

Poultice for Bruises.

Nothing makes so good a poultice for recent bruises as boiled carrots or marshmallows.

Poultice to promote Suppuration.

Indian meal, ...	a sufficient quantity.
Linseed, ...	a handful.
Cayenne, ...	1 tea-spoonful.

To be moistened with boiling vinegar, and applied at the usual temperature.

STYPTICS, TO ARREST BLEEDING.

Witch hazel, (winter bloom,) bark or leaves, 2 ounces.

Make a decoction with the smallest possible quantity of water, and if the bleeding is from the nose, throw it up by means of a syringe; if from the stomach, lungs, or bowels, add more water, and let the animal drink it, and give some by injection.

Styptic to arrest external Bleeding.

Wet a piece of lint with tincture of muriate of iron, and bind it on the part.

There are various other styptics, such as alum water, strong tincture of nutgalls, bloodroot, common salt, fine flour, &c.

ABSORBENTS.

Remarks.—Absorbents are composed of materials partaking of an alkaline character, and are used for the purpose of neutralizing acid matter. The formation of an acid in the stomach arises from some derangement of the digestive organs, sometimes brought on by the improper quantity or quality of the food. It is useless, therefore, to give absorbents, with a view of neutralizing acid, unless the former are combined with tonics, or agents that are capable of restoring the stomach to a healthy state. This morbid state of the stomach is recognized in oxen by a disposition to eat all kinds of trash that comes in their way, such as dirt, litter, &c. They are frequently licking themselves, and often swallow a great deal of hair, which is formed into balls in the stomach and occasions serious irritation. Calves, when fattening, are often fed so injudiciously, that the stomach is incapable of reducing the food to chyme and chyle: the consequence is that a large amount of carbonic acid gas is evolved. Many calves and lambs die from this cause.

A mixture of chalk, saleratus, and soda is often given by farmers; yet they do not afford permanent relief. They do some good by correcting the acidity of the stomach; but the animals are often affected with diarrhœa, or costiveness, loss of appetite, colic, and convulsions. Attention to the diet would probably do more than all the medicine in the world. Yet if they do get sick, something must be done. The best forms of absorbents are the following: they restore healthy action to the lost function at the same time that they neutralize the gas.

FORMS OF ABSORBENTS.

Powdered charcoal, ...	1 table-spoonful.
" snakeroot, ...	half a table-spoonful.
" caraways, ...	1 tea-spoonful.
Hot water, ...	1 quart.

Mix. To be given at one dose, for a cow; half the quantity, or indeed one third, is sufficient for a calf, sheep, or pig.

Another.

Powdered charcoal, ... 1 table-spoonful.

To be given in thoroughwort tea, to which may be added a very small portion of ginger.

Another, adapted to City Use.

Subcarbonate of soda, ...	1 tea-spoonful.
Tincture of gentian, ...	1 ounce.
Infusion of spearmint, ...	1 pint.

Mix. Give a cow the whole at a dose, and repeat daily, for a short time, if necessary. One half the quantity will suffice for a smaller animal.

Drink for Coughs.

Balm of Gilead buds, ...	half an ounce.
Honey, ...	2 table-spoonfuls.
Vinegar, ...	1 wine-glassful.
Water, ...	1 pint

Set the mixture on the fire in an earthen vessel; let it simmer a few minutes. When cool, strain, and it is fit for use. Dose, a wine-glassful, twice a day.

Another.

Balsam copaiba, ...	1 ounce.
Powdered licorice, ...	1 ounce.
Honey, ...	2 table-spoonfuls.
Boiling water, ...	1 quart.

Rub the copaiba, licorice, and honey together in a mortar: after they are well mixed, add the water. Dose, half a pint, night and morning.

Another

Balsam of Tolu, ...	half an ounce.
Powdered marshmallow roots, . . .	1 ounce.
Honey, ...	half a gill.
Boiling water, ...	2 quarts.

Mix. Dose, half a pint, night and morning.

Drink for a Cow after Calving.

Bethwort, ...	1 ounce.
Marshmallows, ...	1 ounce.

First make an infusion of bethwort by simmering it in a quart of water. When cool, strain, and stir in the mallows. Dose half a pint, every two hours.

VETERINARY MATERIA MEDICA,

EMBRACING A LIST OF THE VARIOUS REMEDIES USED BY THE AUTHOR OF THIS WORK IN THE PRACTICE OF MEDICINE ON CATTLE, SHEEP, AND SWINE.

ACACIA, CATECHU, or JAPAN EARTH. It is a powerful astringent and tonic, and given, in half tea-spoonful doses, in mucilage of slippery elm or mallows, is a valuable remedy in diarrhœa, or excessive discharges of urine.

ACACIA GUM makes a good mucilage, and is highly recommended in diseases of the mucous surfaces and urinary organs. It is highly nutritious, and consequently can be given with advantage in locked-jaw.

ACETUM, (vinegar.) This is cooling, and a small portion of it, with an equal quantity of honey, administered in thin gruel, makes an excellent drink in fevers. Diluted with an equal quantity of water, it is employed externally in bruises and sprains. It neutralizes pestilential effluvia, and, combined with capsicum, makes a good application for sore throat.

ACID, PYROLIGNEOUS. This is one of the most valuable articles in the whole *materia medica*. Diluted with equal parts of water, it is applied to ill-conditioned sores and ulcers; it acts as an antiseptic and stimulant. It is obtained from wood by destructive distillation in close vessels. This acid is advantageously applicable to the preservation of animal food. Mr. William Ramsay (*Edinburgh Philosophical Journal*, iii. 21) has made some interesting experiments on its use for this purpose. Herrings and other fish, simply dipped in the acid and afterwards dried in the shade, were effectually preserved, and, when eaten, were found very agreeable to the taste. Herrings slightly cured with salt, by being sprinkled with it for six hours, then drained, next immersed in pyroligneous acid for a few seconds, and afterwards dried in the shade for two months, were found by Mr. Ramsay to be of fine quality and flavor. Fresh beef, dipped in the acid, in the summer season, for the short space of a minute, was perfectly sweet in the following spring. Professor Silliman states, that one quart of the acid added to the common pickle for a barrel of hams, at the time they are laid down, will impart to them the smoked flavor as perfectly as if they had undergone the common process of smoking.

ALDER BARK, BLACK, (*prinos verticillatus.*) A strong decoction makes an excellent wash for diseases of the skin, in all classes of domestic animals.

ALLIUM, (garlic.) This is used chiefly as an antispasmodic. It improves all the secretions, and promotes the function of the skin and kidneys. It is useful also to expel wind and worms. A few kernels may be chopped fine and mixed with the food. When used for the purpose of expelling worms, an ounce of the root should be boiled in a pint of milk, and given in the morning, about an hour before feeding.

ALOES. The best kind is brought from the Island of Socotra, and is supposed to be more safe in its operation than the other kinds. In consequence of the irritative properties of aloes, they are ill adapted to cattle practice; and as a safer article has been recommended, (see *Physic for Cattle,*) we have entirely dispensed with them.

ALTHEA, (marshmallows.) See *Remarks on Poultices.*

ALUM. It possesses powerful astringent properties, and when burnt and pulverized, is useful to remove proud flesh.

AMMONIACUM. Gum ammoniacum is useful for chronic coughs. The dose is two drachms daily, in a quart of gruel.

ANISEED. A good carminative in flatulent colic. The dose is about one ounce, infused in a quart of boiling water.

ANTHEMIS, (camomile.) It is used as a tonic in derangement of the digestive organs, &c. An ounce of the flowers may be infused in a quart of water, and given when cool. It is useful also as an external application in bruises and sprains.

ASH BARK, WHITE. This is a useful remedy in loss of

cud, caused by disease of the liver. Dose, one ounce of the bark, infused in boiling wate When cool, pour off the clear liquor.

Assafœtida. This article is used as an antispasmodic. The dose is from one to two drachms, administered in thin gruel.

Balm, Lemon. See *Fever Drink.*

Balm of Gilead Buds. One cunce of the buds, after being infused in boiling water and strained, makes a good drink for chronic coughs.

Balmony. A good tonic and vermifuge.

Balsam, Canada, is a diuretic, and may be given in slippery elm, in doses of one table-spoonful for diseases of the kidneys.

Balsam of Copaiba, or Capivi, is useful in all diseases of the urinary organs, and, combined with powdered marshmallows and water, makes a good cough drink. Dose, half an ounce.

Balsam of Tolu. Used for the same purpose as the preceding.

Barley. Barley water, sweetened with honey, is a useful drink in fevers.

Bayberry Bark. We have frequently prescribed this article in the preceding pages as an antiseptic and astringent for scouring and dysentery.

Bearberry, (*uva ursi.*) This is a popular diuretic, and is useful when combined with marshmallows. When the urine is thick and deficient in quantity, or voided with difficulty, it may be given in the following form : —

Powdered bearberry, ...	1 ounce.
" marshmallows, ...	2 ounces.
Indian meal, ...	2 pounds.

Mix. Dose, half a pound daily, in the cow's feed.

Bitter Root, (*apocynum androsæmifolium.*) Given in doses of half an ounce of the powdered bark, it acts as an aperient, and is good wherever an aperient is indicated.

Blackberry Root, (*rubus trivialis.*) A valuable remedy for scours in sheep.

Black Root, (*leptandra virginica.*) The extract is used as physic, instead of aloes. (See *Physic for Cattle.*) A strong decoction of the fresh roots will generally act as a cathartic on all classes of animals.

Bloodroot, (*sanguinaria canadensis.*) It is used in our practice as an escharotic. It acts on fungous excrescences, and is a good substitute for nitrate of silver in the dispersion of all morbid growth. One ounce of the powder, infused in boiling vinegar, is a valuable application for rot and mange.

Blue Flag, (*iris versicolor.*) The powdered root is a good vermifuge.

Boneset, (*eupatorium perfoliatum.*) This is a valuable domestic remedy. Its properties are too well known to the farming community to need any description.

Borax. This is a valuable remedy for eruptive diseases of the tongue and mouth. Powdered and dissolved in water, it forms an astringent, antiseptic wash. The usual form of prescription, in veterinary practice, is, —

Powdered borax, ...	half an ounce.
Honey, ...	2 ounces.

Mix.

Buckthorn, (*rhamnus catharticus.*) A sirup made from this plant is a valuable aperient in cattle practice. The dose is from half an ounce to two ounces.

Burdock, (*arctium lappa.*) The leaves, steeped in vinegar, make a good application for sore throat and enlarged glands. The seeds are good to purify the blood, and may be given in the fodder.

Butternut Bark, (*juglans cinerea.*) Extract of butternut makes a good cathartic, in doses of half an ounce. It is much safer than any known cathartic, and, given in doses of two drachms, in hot water, combined with a small quantity of ginger, it forms a useful aperient and alterative. In a constipated habit, attended with loss of cud, it is invaluable. During the American revolution, when medicines were scarce, this article was brought into use by the physicians, and was esteemed by them an excellent substitute for the ordinary cathartics.

CALAMUS, (*acorus calamus.*) A valuable remedy for loss of cud.

CAMOMILE. See *Anthemis*.

CANELLA BARK is an aromatic stimulant, and forms a good stomachic.

CAPSICUM. A pure stimulant. Useful in impaired digestion.

CARAWAY SEED, (*carum carui.*) A pleasant carminative for colic.

CARDAMOM SEEDS. Used for the same purpose as the preceding.

CASSIA BARK, (*laurus cinnamomum.*) Used as a diffusible stimulant in flatulency.

CATECHU, (see ACACIA.)

CATNIP, (*nepeta cataria.*) An antispasmodic in colic.

CEDAR BUDS. An infusion of the buds makes a good vermifuge for sheep and pigs.

CHARCOAL. This is a valuable remedy as an antiseptic for foul ulcers, foot rot, &c.

CLEAVERS, (*galium aparine.*) The expressed juice of the herb acts on the skin and kidneys, increasing their secretions. One tea-spoonful of the juice, given night and morning in a thin mucilage of poplar bark, is an excellent remedy for dropsy, and diseases of the urinary organs. An infusion of the herb, made by steeping one ounce of the leaves and seeds in a quart of boiling water, may be substituted for the expressed juice.

COHOSH, BLACK, (*macrotrys racemosa.*) Useful in dropsy

COLTSFOOT, (*tussilago farfara.*) An excellent remedy for cough.

CRANESBILL, (*geranium maculatum.*) Useful in scours, dysentery, and diarrhœa.

DILL SEED, (*anethum graveolens.*) Its properties are the same as caraways.

DOCK, YELLOW, (*rumex crispus.*) Good for diseases of the liver and of the skin.

ELECAMPANE, (*inula helenium.*) An excellent remedy for cough and asthma, and diseases of the skin.

ELDER FLOWERS, (*sambucus canadensis.*) Used as an aperient for sheep, in constipation.

ELM BARK, (*ulmus fulva.*) This makes a good mucilage. See *Poultices*.

ESSENCE OF PEPPERMINT. Used for flatulent colic. One ounce is the usual dose for a cow. To be given in warm water.

FENNEL SEED. Useful to expel wind.

FERN, MALE, (*aspidium felix mas.*) Used as a remedy for worms.

FLAXSEED. A good lubricant, in cold and catarrh, and in diseases of the mucous surfaces. It makes a good poultice.

FLOWER OF SULPHUR. This is used extensively, in veterinary practice, for diseases of the skin. It is a mild laxative.

FUMIGATIONS. For foul barns and stables, take of

Common salt, ...	4 ounces.
Manganese, ...	1 ounce and a half.

Let these be well mixed, and placed in a shallow earthen vessel; then pour on the mixture, gradually, sulphuric acid, four ounces. The inhalation of the gas which arises from this mixture is highly injurious; therefore, as soon as the acid is poured on, all persons should leave the building, which should immediately be shut, and not opened again for several hours. Dr. White, V. S., says, "This is the only efficacious *fumigation*, it having been found that when glanderous or infectious matter is exposed to it a short time, it is rendered perfectly harmless."

GALBANUM. This gum is used for similar purposes as gum ammoniac and assafœtida.

GALLS. They contain a large amount of tannin, and are powerfully astringent. A strong decoction is useful to arrest hemorrhage.

GARLIC See *Allium*.

GENTIAN. This is a good tonic, and is often employed to remove weakness of the stomach and indigestion.

GINGER. A pure stimulant. Ginger tea is a useful remedy for removing colic and flatulency, and is safer and better adapted to the animal economy, where stimulants are indicated, than alcoholic preparations.

GINSENG, (*panax quinquefolium.*) It possesses tonic and stimulant properties.

GOLDEN SEAL, (*hydrastis canadensis.*) A good tonic, laxative, and alterative.

GOLDTHREAD, (*coptis trifolia.*) A strong infusion of this herb makes a valuable application for eruptions and ulcerations of the mouth. We use it in the following form: —

Goldthread, ...	1 ounce.
Boiling water, ...	1 pint.

Set the mixture aside to cool; then strain, and add a tablespoonful of honey, and bathe the parts twice a day.

GRAINS OF PARADISE. A warming, diffusible stimulant.

HARDHACK, (*spiræa tomentosa.*) Its properties are astringent and tonic. We have used it in cases of "scours" with great success. It is better adapted to cattle practice in the form of extract, which is prepared by evaporating the leaves, stems, or roots. The dose is from one scruple to a drachm for a cow, and from ten grains to one scruple and a half for a sheep, which may be given twice a day, in any bland liquid.

HONEY, (*mel.*) Honey is laxative, stimulant, and nutritious. With vinegar, squills, or garlic, it forms a good cough mixture. Combined with tonics, it forms a valuable gargle, and a detergent for old sores and foul ulcers.

HOPS, (*humulus.*) An infusion of hops is highly recommended in derangement of the nervous system, and for allaying spasmodic twitchings of the extremities. One ounce of the article may be infused in a quart of boiling water, strained, and sweetened with honey, and given, in half pint doses, every four hours. They are used as an external application, in the form of fomentation, for bruises, &c.

HOREHOUND (*marrubium.*) This is a valuable remedy for catarrh and chronic affections of the lungs. It is generally used, in the author's practice, in the following form: An infusion is made in the proportion of an ounce of the herb to a quart of boiling water. A small quantity of powdered marshmallows is then stirred in, to make it of the consistence of thin gruel. The dose is half a pint, night and morning. For sheep and pigs half the quantity will suffice.

HORSEMINT, (*monarda punctata.*) Like other mints, it is antispasmodic and carminative. Useful in flatulent colic.

HORSERADISH. The root scraped and fed to animals laboring under loss of cud, from chronic disease of the digestive organs, and general debility, is generally attended with beneficial results. If beaten into paste with an equal quantity of powdered bloodroot, it makes a valuable application for foul ulcers.

HYSSOP, (*hyssopus officinalis.*) Hyssop tea, sweetened with honey, is useful to promote perspiration in colds and catarrh.

INDIAN HEMP, (*apocynum cannabinum.*) An infusion of this herb acts as an aperient, and promotes the secretions. It may be prepared by infusing an ounce of the powdered or bruised root in a quart of boiling water, which must be placed in a warm situation for a few hours: it should then be strained, and given in half pint doses, at intervals of six hours. A gill of this mixture will sometimes purge a sheep.

INDIGO, WILD, (*baptisia tinctoria.*) We have made some experiments with the inner portion of the bark of this plant, and find it to be very efficacious in the cure of eruptive diseases of the mouth and tongue, lampas, and inflamed gums. A strong decoction (one ounce of the bark boiled for a few minutes in a pint of water) makes a good wash for old sores. A small quantity of powdered slippery elm, stirred into the decoction while hot, makes a good emollient application to sore teats and bruised udder.

JUNIPER BERRIES, (*juniperus.*) These are used in dropsical affections, in conjunction with tonics; also in diseases of the urinary organs.

KINO. This is a powerful astringent, and may be used in

diarrhœa, dysentery, and red water, after the inflammatory symptoms have subsided. We occasionally use it in the following form for red water and chronic dysentery: —

Powdered kino, ...	20 grains.
Thin flour gruel, ...	1 quart.

To be given at a dose, and repeated night and morning, as occasion requires.

LADY'S SLIPPER, (*cypripedum pubescens.*) This is a valuable nervine and antispasmodic, and has been used with great success, in my practice, for allaying nervous irritability. It is a good substitute for opium. It is, however, destitute of all the poisonous properties of the latter. Dose for a cow, half a table-spoonful of the powder, night and morning; to be given in bland fluid.

LICORICE. Used principally to alleviate coughs. The following makes an excellent cough remedy: —

Powdered licorice, ...	1 ounce.
Balsam of Tolu, ...	1 tea-spoonful.
Boiling water, ...	1 quart.

To be given at a dose.

LILY ROOT, (*nymphæa odorata.*) Used principally for poultices.

LIME WATER. This article is used in diarrhœa, and when the discharge of urine is excessive. Being an antacid, it is very usefully employed when cattle are hoven or blown. It is unsafe to administer alone, as it often deranges the digestive organs: it is therefore very properly combined with tonics. The following will serve as an example: —

Lime water, ...	2 ounces.
Infusion of snakehead, (balmony,) . .	2 quarts.

Dose, a quart, night and morning.

LOBELIA, (herb,) (*lobelia inflata.*) This is an excellent antispasmodic. It is used in the form of poultice for locked-jaw, and as a relaxant in rigidity of the muscular structure.

MANDRAKE, (*podophyllum peltatum.*) Used as physic for cattle, (which see.)

MARSHMALLOWS. See *Althea*

MEADOW CABBAGE ROOT, (*ictodes fœtida.*) This plant is used as an antispasmodic in asthma and chronic cough. Dose, a tea-spoonful of the powder, night and morning; to be given in mucilage of slippery elm.

MOTHERWORT, (*leonurus cardiaca.*) A tea of this herb is valuable in protracted labor.

MULLEIN, (*verbascum.*) The leaves steeped in vinegar make a good application for sore throat.

MYRRH. The only use we make of this article, in cattle practice, is to prepare a tincture for wounds, as follows:—

Powdered myrrh, ...	2 ounces.
Proof spirit, ...	1 pint.

Set it aside in a close-covered vessel for two weeks, then strain through a fine sieve, and it is fit for use.

OAK BARK, (*quercus alba.*) A decoction of oak bark is a good astringent, and may be given internally, and also applied externally in falling of the womb or fundament.

OINTMENTS. We have long since discontinued the use of ointments, from a conviction that they do not agree with the flesh of cattle. Marshmallows, or tincture of myrrh, will heal a wound much quicker than any greasy preparation. We have, however, often applied fresh marshmallow ointment to chapped teats, and chafed udder, with decided advantage. It is made as follows: Take of white wax, mutton tallow, and linseed oil, each a pound; marshmallow leaves, two ounces. First melt the wax and tallow, then add the oil, lastly a handful of mallows. Simmer over a slow fire until the leaves are crisp, then strain through a piece of flannel, and stir the mixture until cool.

OLEUM LINI, (flaxseed oil.) This is a useful aperient and laxative in cattle practice, and may be given in all cases of constipation, provided, however, it is not accompanied with chronic indigestion: if such be the case, a diffusible stimulant, combined with a bitter tonic, (golden seal,) aided by an injection, will probably do more good, as they will arouse the digestive function. The above aperient may then be ventured on with safety. The dose for a cow is one pint.

Olive Oil. This is a useful aperient for sheep. The dose is from half a gill to a gill.

Opodeldoc. The different preparations of this article are used for strains and bruises, after the inflammatory action has somewhat subsided.

Liquid Opodeldoc.

Soft soap, ...	6 ounces.
New England rum, ...	1 pint and a half.
Vinegar, ...	half a pint.
Oil of lavender, ...	2 ounces.

The oil of lavender should first be dissolved in an equal quantity of alcohol, and then added to the mixture.

Pennyroyal, (*hedeoma.*) This plant, administered in warm infusion, promotes perspiration, and is good in flatulent colic.

Peppermint, (*mentha piperita.*) An ounce of the herb infused in a quart of boiling water relieves spasmodic pains of the stomach and bowels, and is a good carminative, (to expel wind,) provided the alimentary canal is free from obstruction.

Plantain Leaves, (*plantago major.*) This article is held in high repute for the cure of hydrophobia and bites from poisonous reptiles. The bruised leaves are applied to the parts; the powdered herb and roots to be given internally at discretion.

Pleurisy Root, (*asclepias tuberosa.*) We have given this article a fair trial in cattle practice, and find it to be invaluable in the treatment of catarrh, bronchitis, pleurisy, pneumonia, and consumption. The form in which we generally prescribe it is, —

Powdered pleurisy root, . .	half a table-spoonful.
" marshmallow roots,	1 ounce.

Boiling water sufficient to make a thin mucilage. The

addition of a small quantity of honey increases its diaphoretic properties.

Pomegranate, (*punica granatum.*) The rind of this article is a powerful astringent, and is occasionally used to expel worms. A strong decoction makes a useful wash for falling of the womb, or fundament. Given as an infusion, in the proportion of half an ounce of the rind to a quart of water, it will arrest diarrhœa.

Poplar, (*populus tremuloides.*) It possesses tonic, demulcent, and alterative properties. It is often employed, in our practice, as a local application, in the form of poultice. The infusion is a valuable remedy in general debility, and in cases of diseased urinary organs.

Prince's Pine, (*chimaphila.*) This plant is a valuable remedy in dropsy. It possesses diuretic and tonic properties. It does not produce the same prostration that usually attends the administration of diuretics, for its tonic property invigorates the kidneys, while, at the same time, it increases the secretion of urine. The best way of administering it is by decoction. It is made by boiling four ounces of the fresh-bruised leaves in two quarts of water. After straining, a table-spoonful of powdered marshmallows may be added, to be given in pint doses, night and morning.

Pyroligneous Acid. See *Acid.*

Raspberry Leaves, (*rubus strigosus.*) An infusion of this plant may be employed with great advantage in cases of diarrhœa.

Roman Wormwood, (*ambrosia artemisifolia.*) This plant is a very bitter tonic, and vermifuge. An infusion may be advantageously given in cases of general debility and loss of cud. A strong decoction may be given to sheep and pigs that are infested with worms. If given early in the morning, and before the animals are fed, it will generally have the desired effect.

Rose, Red, (*rosa gallica.*) We have occasionally used the infusion, and find it of great value as a wash for chronic ophthalmia. The infusion is made by pouring a pint of boiling water on a quarter of an ounce of the flowers. It is then strained through fine linen, when it is fit for use.

Sassafras, (*laurus sassafras.*) The bark of sassafras root is stimulant, and possesses alterative properties. We have used it extensively, in connection with sulphur, for eruptive diseases, and for measles in swine, in the following proportions: —

Powdered sassafras,	. . . .	1 ounce.
" sulphur,	. . . .	half a table-spoonful.

Mix, and divide into four parts, one of which may be given, night and morning, in a hot mash.

The pith of sassafras makes a valuable soothing and mucilaginous wash for inflamed eyes.

Senna. A safe and efficient aperient for cattle may be made by infusing an ounce of senna in a quart of boiling water. When cool, strain, then add, manna one ounce, powdered golden seal one tea-spoonful. The whole to be given at a dose.

Skullcap, (*scutellaria lateriflora.*) This is an excellent nervine and antispasmodic. It is admirably adapted to the treatment of locked-jaw, and derangement of the nervous system. An ounce of the leaves may be infused in two quarts of boiling water. After straining, a little honey may be added, and then administered, in pint doses, every four hours.

Snakeroot, Virginia, (*aristolochia serpentaria.*) This article, given by infusion in the proportion of half an ounce of the root to a pint of water, acts as a stimulant and alterative. It is admirably adapted to the treatment of chronic indigestion.

Soap. This article acts on all classes of animals, as a laxative and antacid. It is useful in obstinate constipation of the bowels, in diseases of the liver, and for softening hardened excrement in the rectum. By combining castile soap with butternut, blackroot, golden seal, or balmony, a good aperient is produced, which will generally operate on the bowels in a few hours.

Squill, (*scilla maritima.*) A tea-spoonful of the dried root, given in a thin mucilage of marshmallows, is an excellent remedy for cough, depending on an irritability of the lungs and mucous surfaces.

SULPHUR. This is one of the most valuable articles in the veterinary *materia medica.* It possesses laxative, diaphoretic, and alterative properties, and is extensively employed, both internally and externally, for diseases of the skin. The dose for a cow is a tea-spoonful daily. Its alterative effect may be increased by combining it with sassafras, (which see.)

SUNFLOWER, WILD, (*helianthus divaricatus.*) The seeds of this plant, when bruised and given in any bland fluid, act as a duretic and antispasmodic. Half a table-spoonful of the seeds may be given at a dose, and repeated as occasion requires.

TOLU, BALSAM OF. This balsam is procured by making incisions into the trunk of a tree which flourishes in Tolu and Peru. It has a peculiar tendency to the mucous surfaces, and therefore is very properly prescribed for epizoötic diseases of a catarrhal nature. The dose is half a table-spoonful every night, to be administered in a mucilage of marshmallows. One half the quantity is sufficient for a sheep.

VINEGAR. See *Acetum.*

WITCH HAZEL BARK, (*hamamelis virginica.*) A decoction of this bark is a valuable application for falling of the fundament, or womb. Being a good astringent, an infusion of the leaves is good for scouring in sheep.

WORMSEED, (*chenopodium anthelminticum.*) A tea-spoonful of the powdered seeds, given in a tea of snakeroot, is a good vermifuge: it will, however, require repeated doses, and they should be given at least an hour before the morning meal.

GENERAL REMARKS ON MEDICINES.

HERE, reader, is our *materia medica;* wherein you will find a number of harmless, yet efficient agents, that will, in the treatment of disease, fulfil any and every indication to your entire satisfaction. They act efficiently in the restoration of the diseased system to a healthy state, without producing the slightest injury to the animal economy. The Almighty has furnished us, if we did but know it, a healing balm for every malady to which man and the lower animals are subject. Yet how many of these precious gifts are disregarded for the more popular ones of the chemist! Dr. Brown, professor of botany in the Ohio College, says, "Of the twenty or more thousand species of plants recognized and described by botanists, probably not more than one thousand have ever been used in the art of healing; and not more than one fourth of that number even have a place in our *materia medica* at present. The glorious results, however, attending the researches of those who have preceded us, should inspire us with that confidence and spirit of investigation which will ultimately result in the selection, preparation, and systematic arrangement, of a full, convenient, and efficient *materia medica.*" Unfortunately, the medical fraternity, as well as the farmers, have been accustomed to judge of the power of the remedy by its effects, and not in proportion to its ultimate good. Thus, if a pound of salts be given to a cow, and they produce liquid stools, — in short, "operate well," — they are styled a good medicine, although they leave the mucous surface of the alimentary canal in a weak, debilitated state, and otherwise impair the health; yet this is a secondary consideration. For, if the symptoms of the present malady, for which the salts were given, shall disappear, nothing is thought of the after consequences. The cow may be constipated for several succeeding days, and finally refuse her food; but who suspects that the salts were the cause of it? Who believes that the abstraction of ninety ounces of blood cut short the life of our beloved Washington? We do, and so do others. We are told, in reference to the treatment of a given case, that "the patient will grow worse before he can get better." What makes him worse? The medicine, surely, and nothing else. Now, if ever symptoms are altered, they should be for the better: and if the medicines recommended in this work (provided, however, they are given with ordinary prudence) ever make an animal worse, then we beg of the reader to avoid them as he would a pest-house. This is not all. If any article in this *materia medica*, when given, in the manner we recommend, to an animal in perfect health, shall operate so as to derange such animal's health, — in short, act pathologically, — then it does not deserve a place here, and should not be depended on. But such will not be the result. We recommend farmers to select and preserve a few of these herbs for family use; for they are efficient in the cure of many diseases. And as the services of a physician are not always to be had in small country towns, a little experience in the use and application of simple articles to various diseases seems to be absolutely necessary. It was by the aid of a few of these and similar simple remedies, that we were enabled to preserve the health of the passengers of that ill-fated ship, the Anglo-Saxon. The following testimony has never, until the present time, been made public, and we would not now make use of it, were it not that we wish to show that there are men, and women too, that can appreciate our labors: —

"The undersigned, passengers in the Anglo-Saxon from Boston, feeling it a duty they owe to Dr. G. H. Dadd, surgeon of the ship, would here bear testimony to the valuable medical services and advice rendered by him to us, whilst on shipboard; believing his attendance has been conducive of the greatest benefit; at times almost indispensable, not only during the short passage, but also through the trying period subsequent to the wreck through all of which, the coolness and devotion to the best interests of his employers and of the passengers, exhibited by him, deserve at our hands the highest terms of commendation.

Robert Earle,	A. M. Earle,
S. C. Ames,	Rosálie Pelby,
Benjamin Champney,	Ophelia Anderson,
Lewis Jones,	Helen C. Dove,
Hamilton G. Wild,	Eleanor Teresa McIver,
W. A. Barnes,	John Hills,
Gideon D. Scull,	Frances Blenkam,
W. Allan Gay,	Harriet Phillips,
Isaac Jenkins,	Louisa A. Bigelow
Prescott Bigelow,	

Eastport, May 9 1847."

Notwithstanding this disaster, Enoch Train, Esq., of Boston, with a liberality which does him credit, appointed us surgeon of the ship Mary Ann, commanded by Captain Albert Brown; thus giving us a second opportunity of proving what we had asserted, viz., *that the emigrants might be brought to the United States in better condition, and with less deaths, than had heretofore been done.* It must be remembered that about this time the typhus, or ship fever, was making sad havoc amongst all classes of men, and many talented professional men fell victims to the dire malady. We left Liverpool at a sickly season, having on board two hundred persons, and were fortunate enough to land them in this city, all in good health. Several ships which sailed at the same time, bound also to different ports in the United States, lost, on the passage, from ten to twenty persons, although each ship was furnished with a medical attendant. Here, then, is a proof that our agents cure while others fail.

PROPERTIES OF PLANTS.

Professor Curtis tells us that "herbs, during their growth, preserve their medicinal properties, commencing at the root, and continuing upward, through the stem and leaves, to the flowers and seeds, until fully grown. When the root begins to die, the properties ascend from it towards the seed, where, at last, they are the strongest. Even the virtues of the leaves, after they get their full growth, often go into the seed, which will not be so well developed if the leaves are plucked off early; as corn fills and ripens best when the leaves are left on the stalks till they die. In the annual and biennial plants, the root is worthless after the seed is ripe, and the stem also is of very little value; what virtue there is residing in the bark and leaves also lose their properties as fast as they lose their freshness. All leaves and stems that have lost their color, or become shrivelled, while the roots are in the earth, have lost much of their medicinal power, and should be rejected from medicine." Seeds and fruit should be gathered when ripe or fully matured.

Flowers should be gathered just at the time they come into bloom.

Leaves should be gathered when they have arrived at their full growth, are green, and full of the juices of the plant. Barks should be gathered as early in the spring as they will peal.

Roots should be gathered in the fall, after they have perfectly matured, or early in the spring, before they commence germinating and growing.

POTATO.

Boiled potatoes, mixed up with steamed cornstalks, shorts, &c., make an excellent compound for fattening cattle; yet, at the present time, they are too expensive for general use. We hope, however, that ere long our farmers will take hold of this subject in good earnest, — we allude to the causes of potato rot, — and restore this valuable article of food to its original worth. A few remarks on this subject seem to be called for.

Remarks on the Potato Rot.

Where are the fine, mealy, substantial "apples of the earth" gone? — and Echo answers, "Where?" They are not to be found at the present day. The farmers have suffered great losses, in some instances by a partial, and in others by a total, failure of their crops. Numberless experiments have been tried to prevent this great national calamity, yet they have all proved abortive, for the simple reason that we have been only treating the symptoms, while the disease has taken a firmer hold, and hurried our subjects to a premature decay.

Different theories have been suggested with a view of explaining the causes of the potato rot, none of which are satisfactory. We have the "fungous theory," "insect theory," "moisture theory," "theory of *degeneration*," and "the chemical theory of defective elements." In relation to the "fungous theory" we observe that fungi inhabit decaying organic bodies. They are considered to be a common pest to all kinds of plants, like parasites, living at the expense of those plants. We do not expect to find fungi in good healthy vegetables, at least while they possess a high grade of vital action. It is only when morbid deposits and chemical agencies overcome the integrity or vital affinity of the vegetable that fungous growth commences.

In the fungous development, the living parts of the vegetable are not always destroyed; yet these fungi obstruct vital action by their deposits or accumulations; hence the small vessels that lead from centre to surface are partly paralyzed, and the power peculiar to all vegetables of throwing off useless or excrementitious matter is intercepted. This is not all. The process of imperceptible elimination, which might restore the balance of power in any thing like a vigorous plant, is thus impaired.

Now, it is evident that the fungi are not the cause of the potato rot; they are only the mere effects, the symptoms: preceding these were other manifestations of disorder, and these manifestations, in their different grades, might with equal propriety be charged as causes of the potato rot. The deterioration of the potato has been going on in a gradual manner for a long time. A mild form of disease has existed for a number of years, making such imperceptible change that it has escaped the observation of many until late years, when the article became so unpalatable that our attention has been called to it in good earnest; and by the aid of the microscope we have discovered the fungi. Has this discovery benefited the agriculturist? Not a particle.

The theory of degeneration, without doubt, will assist us to explain the why and wherefore of the potato rot. But this is not all; the community want to know the cause of this degeneracy. We have spent some time in the investigation of this subject, and now give the public, in a condensed form, our opinion of this matter. We may err, but our progress is towards the full discovery of the *direct cause*, and the ways and means best adapted to prevent this sad calamity. The potato came into existence at a certain period in the history of the world. After its discovery, it was taken from the mother soil, the land of its nativity, planted in different parts of the world and grew to apparent perfection. Our opinion is, that the transplanting was one of the causes of this degeneracy. It is generally known that indigenous plants do not thrive so well on foreign soil as in their native; for example, the plants of the sunny south cannot be made to flourish here in the same degree of perfection as at the south; they require the genial warmth of the sun's rays, which our northern climates lack. The soil, too, must be adapted to each particular plant. It is true we do cultivate them by ingenuity and chemical agency; yet they seldom equal the original. Need we ask the farmer if he can, from the soil of New England, produce a St. Michael orange equal to one grown on its native soil? or if a squash will grow in the deserts of Arabia? All vegetables, as well as animals, possess a certain amount of vital power, which enables them to resist, to a certain degree, all encroachments on their healthy operations. The potato, having been deprived, in some measure, of its essential element, lost its reciprocal equilibrium, and has ever since been a prey to whatever destructive agents may be present, whether they exist in the soil or atmosphere. Yet we conceive that its total destruction is dependent on another cause, which has been entirely overlooked; for, in spite of the gradual deterioration alluded to, the potato will, for a number of years, continue to keep up a low form of vitality and result in something like a potato. In order to comprehend the subject, let us, for a moment, consider the conditions necessary for the germination and perfection of vegetable bodies. We shall then be able to decide as to whether or no we have complied with such conditions. The first condition is, we must have *a perfect germ;* secondly, *a ripe seed;* and lastly, *nutrimental agents in the soil, composed of carbon, hydrogen, and oxygen.*

The potato requires but a small quantity of moisture to develop the germinating principle; for we have every day evidences of its ability to send forth its fibres, even in the open air. Now, the premature development of these fibrous radicles, or roots, debilitates the tuber; in short, we have a sick potato. Is the potato, under such circumstances, a perfect germ? No. If you examine the potato, with its roots and stem, you will find the cutis, or skin, and mucous membrane. This external skin, *including that of plant, stalk, leaf, and ball,* is to the potato what the skin and lungs are to animals; they, each of them, absorb atmospheric food, and throw off excrementitious matter; the roots and fibres are to the vegetable what the alimentary canal is to the animal. A large portion of the food of vegetables is found in the soil, and enters the vegetable system, through its capillary circulation, by the process of imperceptible elimination and absorption. Now, you must bear in mind that the fibres, stem, and leaves are delicate and tender organs; they are studded with millions of little pores, covered with a membrane of delicate texture, easily lacerated. When these delicate organs are rudely torn off or lacerated, the potato immediately gives evidence of the encroachments of disease; it shrinks, withers, and, although the soil abounds in all that is necessary for its growth and future development, it is not in a fit state to carry on the chemico-vital process. We often take the potato from the soil with a view of preserving it for seed, without any definite knowledge of the exact time of its maturity; as the season arrives for again replanting, the fibres are torn off, and the potato itself is often cut up into two or three pieces; sometimes, however, the smaller potatoes are used for seed. Both practices are open to strong objection Oftentimes the cut surfaces of the potato are exposed to atmospheric air; evaporation commences, they lose their firm texture, and are more fit for swine than for planting.

The cause of the total destruction may exist in a loss of polarity! We know that all organic and inorganic bodies are subject to the laws of electricity — each has its polarity. Men who are engaged in mining can testify that the stratification of the earth is alternately negative and positive. The hemispheres of the earth are also governed by the same law; for, if you take a magnetic needle and toss it up in this hemisphere, which is negative, the positive end will come to the ground first; but if you pass the magnetic equator, which crosses the common equator in 23° 28′, and then toss the needle up, its negative end will fall downwards. Hence we infer that the potato has a polarity, just as man has; and this is the reason of their definite character. Take a bean, and destroy its polarity by cutting it into several pieces, as you do the potato, and all the men on earth cannot make it germinate and grow to perfection. It will die just as a man will, if you destroy the polarity of his brain by wounding it.

Take an egg, and destroy its polarity by making a small puncture through it, and you can never get a chicken from it. A man or an animal will die of locked-jaw, caused by a splinter entering the living organism; and why? Because their electrical equilibrium, or their polarity, is destroyed. Some of our readers may desire to know how we can prove that electricity plays a part in the germination and growth of animals and vegetables. In verification of it, we will give a few examples. A dish of salad may, by the aid of electricity, be raised in an hour. Hens' eggs can be hatched by a similar process in a few hours, which would require many days by animal heat. By the aid of electricity, water, which consists of oxygen and hydrogen, may be decomposed, and its elements set free. The poles of a galvanic battery may be applied to a dead body, and that body made to imitate the functions of life.

And lastly, it is through the medium of electrical attraction which bodies have for each other, that all the chemical compositions and decompositions depend. Bodies must be in opposite states of electricity in order to produce a result. Now, if the polarity of the potato is destroyed in the manner we have just alluded to, or should it be destroyed by coming in contact with the blade of a knife, *the latter conducting off the electrical current*, or by any other means, it must deteriorate. We are told that "the potato has several germinating points, and that a part will grow just as well as the whole." Such reasoning will not stand the test of common experience.

For example: the Almighty has endowed man with various faculties, and the perfection of his organism depends on these faculties, as a whole. Now, he may lose a leg, and yet be capable of performing the ordinary duties of life; but this does not prove that he might not perform them much better with both legs. So in reference to the potato. The fact of its ability to reproduce its kind from a small portion of the whole — a mere bud — should not satisfy us that a perfect germ is unnecessary. Then the question arises, How shall we restore the original identity of this valuable article of food?

We have, in the early part of this work, recommended the farmers to study the laws of vegetable physiology. This will furnish them with the right kind of information. We would, however, suggest to those who are desirous of making experiments, to comply with the conditions already alluded to, viz., plant a perfect germ, by which means the potato may be improved. Yet, in order to restore its identity, we must commence by germinating from the seed, and plant that on soil abounding in the constituents necessary for its development. Elevated land abounding in small stones, and hill sides facing the south, are the best situations. Potatoes should never be cultivated on the same spot for two successive years.

In relation to the insect theory, we would observe, that it throws no light on the cause of the potato rot; for, in its

14*

gradual decay, that vegetable undergoes various changes; the particles of which it is composed assume new forms, and enter into new combinations; its elementary substances are separated, giving birth to new compounds, some of which result in an insect. We all know that animal and vegetable bodies may remain in a state of putrefaction in water, and be dissolved in the dust; yet some of their original atoms appear in a new system. Hence the insect theory has no more to do with the cause of the potato rot than the fungus.

TREATMENT OF DISEASE IN DOGS.

PRELIMINARY REMARKS.

A GOOD watch dog is of inestimable value to the farmer; and as very little is at present understood of the nature and treatment of their maladies, we have thought that a few general directions would be acceptable, not only to the farmer, but to every man who loves a dog. We have paid considerable attention to the treatment of disease in this class of animals, and have generally found that most of their maladies will yield very readily to our sanative agents. Most of the remedies recommended by *allopathic* writers for dogs, like those recommended for horses and cattle, would at any time destroy the animal; consequently, if it ever recovers, it does so in spite of the violence done to the constitution. We hope to rescue the dog, as well as other classes of domestic animals, from a cruel system of medication; for this we labor, and to this work our life is devoted. We ask the reader to take into consideration the destructive nature of the articles used on these faithful animals. Some of them are the most destructive poisons that can be found in the whole world. For example, several authors recommend, in the treatment of disease in the canine race, the following:—

Tartar emetic, a very few grains of which will kill a man — yet recommended for dogs.

Calomel, a very fashionable remedy, used for producing ulcerated gums and for rotting the teeth of thousands of the human family, as the dentists can testify. Not fit for a dog, yet prescribed by most dog fanciers.

Lunar caustic, recommended by Mr. Lawson for fits; to be given internally with cobwebs!! Our opinion is, that it would be likely to give any four-footed creature "*fits*" that took it.

Cowhage, corrosive sublimate, tin-filings, sugar of lead, white precipitate, oil of turpentine, opium, nitre—these, together with aloes, jalap, tobacco, hellebore, and a very small proportion of sanative agents, make up the list. In view of the great destruction that is likely to attend the administration of these and kindred articles, we have substituted others, which may be given with safety. Why should the poor dog be compelled to swallow down such powerful and destructive agents? He is entitled to better treatment, and we flatter ourselves that wherever these pages shall be read, he will receive it. In reference to the value of dogs, Mr. Lawson says, "Independent of his beauty, vivacity, strength, and swiftness, he has the interior qualities that must attract the attention and esteem of mankind. Intelligent, humble, and sincere, the sole happiness of his life seems to be to execute his master's commands. Obedient to his owner, and kind to all his friends, to the rest he is indifferent. He knows a stranger by his clothes, his voice, or his gestures, and generally forbids his approach with marks of indignation. At night, when the guard of the house is committed to his care, he seems proud of the charge; he continues a watchful sentinel, goes his rounds, scents strangers at a distance, and by barking gives them notice that he is on duty; if they attempt to break in, he becomes fiercer, threatens, flies at them, and either conquers alone, or alarms those who have more interest in coming to his assistance. The flock and herd are even more obedient to the dog than to the shepherd: he conducts them, guards them, and keeps them from capriciously seeking danger; and their enemies he considers as his own."

DISTEMPER.

Symptoms. — If the animal is a watch dog, (such are usually confined in the daytime,) the person who is in the daily habit of feeding him will first observe a loss of appetite; the animal will appear dull and lazy; shortly after, there is a watery discharge from the eyes and nose, resembling that which accompanies catarrh. As the disease advances, general debility supervenes, accompanied with a weakness of the hind extremities. The secretions are morbid; for example, some are constipated, and pass high-colored urine; others are suddenly attacked with diarrhœa, scanty urine, and vomiting. Fits are not uncommon during the progress of the disease.

Treatment. — If the animal is supposed to have eaten any improper food, we commence the treatment by giving an emetic.

Emetic for Dogs.

Powdered lobelia, (herb,)	1 tea-spoonful.
Warm water, ...	1 wine-glass.

Mix, and administer at a dose.

(A table-spoonful of common salt and water will generally vomit a dog.)

If this dose does not provoke emesis, it should not be repeated, for it may act as a relaxant, and carry the morbid accumulations off by the alimentary canal. If the bowels are constipated, use injections of soap-suds. If the symptoms are complicated, the following medicine must be prepared:

Powdered mandrake, ...	1 table-spoonful.
" sulphur, ...	1 tea-spoonful.
" charcoal, ...	2 tea-spoonfuls.
" marshmallows, . . .	1 table-spoonful.

Mix. Divide the mass into six parts, and administer one in honey night and morning, for the first day; after which a single powder, daily, will suffice. The diet to consist of mush, together with a drink of thin arrowroot. If, however, the animal be in a state of plethora, very little food should be given him.

If the strength fails, support it with beef tea. Should a diarrhœa attend the malady, give an occasional drink of hardhack tea.

FITS.

Dogs are subject to epileptic fits, which are often attended with convulsions. They attack dogs of all ages, and under every variety of management. Dogs that are apparently healthy are often suddenly attacked. The nervous system of the dog is very susceptible to external agents; hence whatever raises any strong passion in them often produces fits. Pointers and setters have often been known to suffer an attack during the excitement of the chase. Fear will also produce fits; and bitches, while suckling, if burdened with a number of pups, and not having a sufficiency of nutriment to support the lacteal secretion, often die in convulsive fits. Young puppies, while teething, are subject to fits: simply scarifying their gums will generally give temporary relief. Lastly, fits may be hereditary, or they may be caused by derangement of the stomach. In all cases of fits, it is very necessary, in order to treat them with success, that we endeavor, as far as possible, to ascertain the causes, and remove them as far as lies in our power: this accomplished, the cure is much easier.

Treatment. — Whenever the attack is sudden and violent, and the animal is in good flesh, plunge him into a tub of warm water, and give an injection of the same, to which a tea-spoonful of salt may be added. It is very difficult, in fact improper, to give medicine during the fit; but as soon as it is over, give

Manna, ...	1 tea-spoonful.
Common salt, ...	half a tea-spoonful.

Add a small quantity of water, and give it at a dose.

Another.

Make an infusion of mullein leaves, and give to the amount of a wine-glass every four hours. With a view of preventing a recurrence of fits, keep the animal on a vegetable diet. If the bowels are constipated, give thirty grains of extract of butternut, or, if that cannot be readily procured, substitute an infusion of senna and manna, to which a few caraways may be added.

If the nervous system is deranged, which may be known by the irritability attending it, then give a tea-spoonful of the powdered nervine, (lady's slipper.) The diet must consist of boiled articles, and the animal must be allowed to take exercise.

WORMS.

Worms may proceed from various causes; but they are seldom found in healthy dogs. One of the principal causes is debility in the digestive organs.

Indications of Cure. — To tone up the stomach and other organs, — by which means the food is prevented from running into fermentation, — and administer vermifuges. The following are good examples: —

Oil of wormseed, ...	1 tea-spoonful.
Powdered assafœtida, ...	30 grains.

To be given every morning fasting. Two doses will generally suffice

Another.

Powdered mandrake, . . .	half a table-spoonful.
Virginia snakeroot,	1 tea-spoonful.

Divide into four doses, and give one every night, in honey

Another.

Make an infusion of the sweet fern, (*comptonea asplenifolia*,) and give an occasional drink, followed by an injection of the same.

Another.

Powdered golden seal, . . .	half a table-spoonful.
Common brown soap, . . .	1 ounce.

Rub them well together in a mortar, and form the mass into pills about the size of a hazel-nut, and give one every night.

MANGE.

This disease is too well known to need any description. The following are deemed the best cures: —

External Application for Mange.

Powdered charcoal, ...	half a table-spoonful.
" sulphur, ...	1 ounce.

Soft soap sufficient to form an ointment.

To be applied externally for three successive days; at the end of which time, the animal is to be washed with castile soap and warm water, and afterwards wiped dry.

The internal remedies consist of equal parts of sulphur and cream of tartar, half a tea-spoonful of which may be given daily, in honey.

When the disease becomes obstinate, and large, scabby eruptions appear on various parts of the body, take

Pyroligneous acid, ...	2 ounces.
Water, ...	1 pint.

Wash the parts daily, and keep the animal on a light diet.

INTERNAL ABSCESS OF THE EAR.

In this complaint, the affected side is generally turned downwards, and the dog is continually shaking his head.

Treatment. — In the early stages, foment the part twice a day with an infusion of marshmallows. As soon as the abscess breaks, wash with an infusion of raspberry leaves, and if a watery discharge continues, wash with an infusion of white oak bark.

ULCERATION OF THE EAR.

External ulcerations should be washed twice a day with

Pyroligneous acid, ...	2 ounces.
Water, ...	8 ounces.

Mix.

As soon as the ulcerations assume a healthy appearance, touch them with Turlington's balsam or tincture of gum catechu.

INFLAMMATION OF THE BOWELS.

Whenever inflammation of the bowels makes its appearance, it is a sure sign that there is a loss of equilibrium in the circulation, and this disturbance may arise from a col lapse of the external surface, or from irritation produced by hardened excrement on the mucous membrane of the intestines. An attack is recognized by acute pain in the abdominal region. The dog gives signs of suffering when moved and the bowels are generally constipated.

Treatment. — Endeavor to equalize the circulation by putting the animal into a warm bath, where he should remain about five minutes. When taken out, the surface must be rubbed dry. Then give the following injection: —

Linseed oil, ...	4 ounces.
Warm water, ...	1 gill.

Mix.

To allay the irritation of the bowels, give the following: —

Powdered pleurisy root, . . .	1 tea-spoonful.
" marshmallow root, . .	1 table-spoonful.

Mix, and divide into three parts; one to be given every four hours.

Should vomiting be a predominant symptom, a small quantity of saleratus, dissolved in spearmint tea, may be given.

Should not this treatment give relief, make a fomentation of hops, and apply it to the belly; and give half an ounce of manna. The only articles of food and drink should consist of barley gruel and mush. If, however, the dog betrays great heat, thirst, panting, and restlessness, a small quantity of cream of tartar may be added to the barley gruel. The bath and clysters may be repeated, if necessary.

INFLAMMATION OF THE BLADDER.

This requires the same treatment as the preceding malady

ASTHMA.

Dogs that are shut up in damp cellars, and deprived of pure air and exercise, are frequently attacked with asthma. Old dogs are more liable to asthma than young ones.

Treatment. — Endeavor to ascertain the cause, and remove it. Let the animal take exercise in the open air. The diet to consist of cooked vegetables; a small quantity of boiled meat may be allowed; raw meat should not be given.

Compound for Asthma.

Powdered bloodroot, . . .	of each, 1 tea-spoonful.
" lobelia, ...	
" marshmallows, .	
" licorice, . . .	

Mix. Divide into twelve parts, and give one night and morning. If they produce retching, reduce the quantity of lobelia. The object is not to vomit, but to induce a state of nausea or relaxation.

PILES.

Piles are generally brought on by confinement, over-feeding, &c., and show themselves by a red, sore, and protruded rectum. Dogs subject to constipation are most likely to be attacked.

Treatment. — Give the animal half a tea-spoonful of sulphur for two or three mornings, and wash the parts with an infusion of white oak bark. If they are very painful, wash two or three times a day with an infusion of hops, and keep the animal on a light diet.

DROPSY.

Dropsy is generally preceded by loss of appetite, cough diminution of natural discharge of urine, and costiveness. The abdomen shortly afterwards begins to enlarge.

Treatment. — It is sometimes necessary to evacuate the fluid by puncturing the abdomen; but this will seldom avail much unless the general health is improved, and the suppressed secretions restored. The following is the best remedy we know of: —

Powdered flagroot, ...	of each a quarter of an ounce.
" male fern, . . .	
Scraped horseradish, ...	a tea-spoonful.

Mix. Divide into eight parts, and give one night and morning. Good nutritious diet must be allowed.

SORE THROAT.

A strong decoction of mullein leaves applied to a sore throat will seldom fail in curing it.

SORE EARS.

A dog's ears may become sore and scabby from being torn, or otherwise injured. In such cases, they should be anointed with marshmallow ointment.

SORE FEET.

If the feet become sore from any disease between the claws, apply a poultice composed of equal parts of marshmallows and charcoal; after which the following wash will complete the cure: —

Pyroligneous acid, ...	1 ounce.
Water, ...	6 ounces.

Mix, and wash with a sponge twice a day.

WOUNDS.

Turlington's Balsam is the best application for wounds. Should a dog be bitten by one that is mad, give him a teaspoonful of lobelia in warm water, and bind some of the same article on the wound.

SPRAINS.

For sprains of any part of the muscular structure, use one of the following prescriptions: —

Oil of wormwood, ...	1 ounce.
Tincture of lobelia, ...	2 ounces.
Infusion of hops, ...	1 quart.

Mix. Bathe the part twice a day.

Another.

Wormwood, ...	of each a handful.
Thoroughwort, ...	of each a handful.
New England rum, ...	1 pint.

Set them in a warm place for a few hours, then bathe the part with the liquid; and bind some of the herb on the part, if practicable.

SCALDS.

If a dog be accidentally scalded, apply, with as little delay as possible, —

Lime water, ...	equal parts.
Linseed oil, ...	

OPHTHALMIA.

Ophthalmia is supposed to be contagious; yet a mild form may result from external injury, as blows, bruises, or extraneous bodies introduced under the eyelid. The eye is such a delicate and tender organ, that the smallest particle of any foreign body lodging on its surface will cause great pain and swelling.

Treatment. — Take a tea-spoonful of finely-pulverized marshmallow root, add sufficient hot water to make a thin mucilage, and with this wash the eye frequently. Keep the animal in a dark place, on a light diet; and if the eyes are very red and tender, give a pill composed of twenty-nine grains extract of butternut and ten grains cream of tartar.

If a purulent discharge sets in, bathe the eye with infusion of camomile or red rose leaves, and give the following: —

Powdered pleurisy root, ...	equal parts.
" bloodroot, ...	
" sulphur, ...	

Dose, half a table-spoonful daily. To be given in honey. When the eyelids adhere together, wash with warm milk.

WEAK EYES.

It often happens that, after an acute attack, the eyes are left in a weak state, when there is a copious secretion of fluid continually running from them. In such cases the eyes may be washed, night and morning, with pure cold water, and the general health must be improved: for the latter purpose, the following preparation is recommended: —

Manna, ...	1 ounce.
Powdered gentian, ...	1 tea-spoonful.
" mandrake, ...	half a tea-spoonful.

Rub them together in a mortar, and give a pill, about the size of a hazel-nut, every night. If the manna is dry, a little honey will be necessary to amalgamate the mass.

FLEAS AND VERMIN.

Fleas and vermin are very troublesome to dogs; yet they may easily be got rid of by bathing the dog with an infusion of lobelia for two successive mornings, and afterwards washing with water and castile soap.

HYDROPHOBIA.

Whenever one dog is bitten by another, and the latter is supposed to labor under this dreadful malady, immediate steps should be taken to arrest it; for a dog once bitten by another, whatever may be the stage or intensity of the disease, is never safe. The disease may appear in a few days; in some instances, it is prolonged for eight months.

Symptoms.—Mr. Lawson tells us that "the first symptom appears to be a slight failure of the appetite, and a disposition to quarrel with other dogs. A total loss of appetite generally succeeds. A mad dog will not cry out on being struck, or show any sign of fear on being threatened. In the height of the disorder, he will bite all other dogs, animals, or men. When not provoked, he usually attacks only such as come in his way; but, having no fear, it is very dangerous to strike or provoke him. The eyes of mad dogs do not look red or fierce, but dull, and have a peculiar appearance, not easy to be described. Mad dogs seldom bark, but occasionally utter a most dismal and plaintive howl, expressive of extreme distress, and which they who have once heard can never forget. They do not froth at the mouth; but their lips and tongue appear dry and foul, or slimy. They cannot swallow water.' Mr. Lawson, and indeed many veterinary practitioners, have come to the conclusion that all remedies are fallacious! *

Remarks.—In White's Dictionary we are informed that the tops of yellow broom have been used for hydrophobia in the human subject with great success; and we do not hesitate to say that they might be used with equal success on beasts. Dr. Muller, of Vienna, has lately published, in the *Gazette de Santé*, some facts which go to show that the yellow broom is invaluable in the treatment of this malady. Dr. White tells us that "M. Marochetti gave a decoction of yellow broom to twenty-six persons who had been bitten by a mad dog, viz., nine men, eleven women, and six children. Upon an examination of their tongues, he discovered pimples in five men, three children, and in all the women. The seven

* They probably only allude to cauterization, cutting out the bitten part, and the use of poisons. It cannot be expected that such processes and agents should ever cure the disease. Let them try our agents before they pronounce "all remedies fallacious." Let them try the *alisma plantago*, (plantain,) yellow broom tops, *scutellaria* (skullcap,) lobelia, Greek valerian, &c

that were free from pimples took the decoction of broom six weeks and recovered."

The same author informs us that "M. Marochetti, during his residence at Ukraine, in the year 1813, attended fifteen persons who had been bitten by a mad dog. While he was making preparations for cauterizing the wounds, some old men requested him to treat the unfortunate people according to the directions of a peasant in the neighborhood, who had obtained great reputation for the cure of hydrophobia. The peasant gave to fourteen persons, placed under his care, a strong decoction of the yellow broom; he examined, twice a day, the under part of the tongue, where he had generally discovered little pimples, containing, as he supposed, the hydrophobic poison. These pimples at length appeared, and were observed by M. Marochetti himself. As they formed, the peasant opened them, and cauterized the parts with a red hot needle; after which the patients gargled with the same decoction. The result of this treatment was, that the fourteen patients returned cured, having drank the decoction six weeks." The following case will prove the value of the plantain, (*plantago major.*) We were called upon, October 25, 1850, to see a dog, the property of Messrs. Stewart & Forbes, of Boston. From the symptoms, we were led to suppose that the animal was in the incipient stage of canine madness. We directed him to be securely fastened, kept on a light diet, &c. The next day, a young Newfoundland pup was placed in the cellar with the patient, who seized the little fellow, and crushed his face and nose in a most shocking manner, both eyes being almost obliterated. The poor pup lingered in excruciating torment until the owner, considering it an act of charity, had it killed. This act of ferocity on the part of the patient confirmed our suspicions as to the nature of the malady. We commenced the treatment by giving him tea-spoonful doses of powdered plantain, (*plantago major,*) night and morning, in the food, and in the course of a fortnight, the eye (which, during the early stage of the malady, had an unhealthy appearance) assumed its natural state, and the appetite returned; in short, the dog got rapidly well. We feel confident that, if this case had been neglected, it might have terminated in canine madness.

We are satisfied that the plantain possesses valuable anti septic and detergent properties. Dr. Beach tells us that "a negro at the south obtained his freedom by disclosing a nostrum for the bites of snakes, the basis of which was the plantain." A writer states that a toad, in fighting with a spider, as often as it was bitten, retired a few steps, ate of the plantain, and then renewed the attack. The person deprived it of the plant, and it soon died.

Treatment. — Let the suspected dog be confined by himself, so that he cannot do injury. Then take two ounces of lobelia, and one ounce of sulphur, place them in a common wash tub, and add several gallons of boiling water. As soon as it is sufficiently cool, plunge the dog into it, and let him remain in it several minutes. Then give an infusion of either of the following articles: yellow broom, plantain, or Greek valerian, one ounce of the herb to a pint of water. An occasional tea-spoonful of the powdered plantain may be allowed with the food, which must be entirely vegetable. If the dog has been bitten, wash the part with a strong infusion of lobelia, and bind some of the herb on the part. The treatment should be continued for several days, or until the animal recovers, and all danger is past.

(For information on the causes of madness, the reader is referred to my work on the Horse, p. 108.)

MALIGNANT MILK SICKNESS OF THE WESTERN STATES, OR CONTAGIOUS TYPHUS.

THIS name applies to a disease said to be very fatal in the Western States, attacking certain kinds of live stock, and also persons who make use of the meat and dairy products of such cattle.

The cause, nature, and treatment of this disease is so little understood among medical men, and such an alarming mortality attends their practice, that many of the inhabitants of the west and south-west depend entirely on their domestic remedies. "It is in that country emphatically one of the *opprobria medicorum*." Nor are the mineralites any more successful in the treatment of other diseases incidental to the Great West. Their Peruvian bark, *quinine,* and calomel, immense quantities of which are used without any definite knowledge of their *modus operandi,* fail in a great majority of cases. If they were only to substitute powdered charcoal and sulphur for calomel, both in view of prevention and cure, aided by good nursing, then the mortality would be materially diminished. The success attending the treatment of upwards of sixty cases of yellow fever, by Mrs. Shall, the proprietress of the City Hotel, New Orleans, only one of which proved fatal, is attributed to good nursing. She knew nothing of blood-letting, calomelizing, or narcotizing. The same success attended the practice of Dr. A. Hunn, of Kentucky, in the treatment of typhus fever, (which resembles milk sickness,) who cured every case by plunging his patients immediately into a hot bath.

"The whole indication of cure in this disease is to bring on reaction, to recall the poison which is mixed with the blood and thrown to the centre, which can only be done by inducing a copious perspiration in the most prompt and energetic manner. If I mistake not, where sweating was produced in this complaint, recovery invariably followed, while bleeding, mercury, &c., only aggravated it."

From such facts as these, as well as from numerous others we may learn, that disease is not under the control of the boasted science of medicine, as practised by our allopathic brethren. Many millions of animals, as well as members of the human family, have died from a misapplication of medicine, and officious meddling.

The destruction that in former years attended milk sickness may be learned from the fact, that in the western settlements, its prevalence often served as a cause to disband a community, and compel the inhabitants to seek a location which enjoyed immunity from its occurrence. The legislatures of several of the Western States have offered rewards for the discovery of the origin of the milk sickness. No one that we know of has ever yet claimed the reward. In view of the great lack of information on this subject, we freely contribute our mite, which may serve, in some degree, to dispel the impenetrable mystery by which it is surrounded.

We shall first show that it is not produced by the atmosphere alone, which by some is supposed to be the cause.

"It is often found to occupy an isolated spot, comprehending an area of one hundred acres, whilst for a considerable distance around it is not produced."

If the disease had its sole origin in the atmosphere, it would not be thus confined to a certain location; for every one knows, that the gentlest zephyr would waft the enemy into the surrounding localities, and there the work of destruction would commence. The reader is probably aware that bodies whose specific gravity exceeds that of air, such as grass, seeds, &c., are conveyed through that medium from one field to another. The miasma of epidemics is said to be conveyed from one district to another "on the wings of the wind." Hence, if milk sickness was of atmospheric or even epidemic origin, it would prevail in adjoining states. This is not the case; for we are told that "this fatal disease seldom, if ever, prevails westward of the Alleghany Mountains or in the bordering states."

The atmosphere which surrounds this globe was intended

by the divine Artist for the purpose of respiration, and it is well adapted to that purpose: it cannot be considered a pathological agent, or a cause of disease. In crowded assemblies, and in close barns and stables, it may hold in solution noxious gases, which, as we have already stated in different parts of this work, are injurious to the lungs; but as regards the atmosphere itself, in an uncontaminated state, it is a physiological agent. It always preserves its identity, and is always represented by the same equivalents of oxygen, nitrogen, and carbonic acid gas. Liebig says, "One hundred volumes of air have been found, at every period and in every climate, to contain twenty-one volumes of oxygen."

Thus oxygen and nitrogen unite in certain equivalents: the result is atmospheric air; and they cannot be made to unite in any other proportions. Suppose the oxygen to be in excess, what would be the result? A universal conflagration would commence; the hardest rocks, and even the diamond, (considered almost indestructible,) would melt with "fervent heat." If, on the other hand, nitrogen was in excess, then every living thing, including both animal and vegetable, would instantly die. Hence we infer that the atmosphere cannot be considered as the cause of this disease.

Causes. — A creeping vine has been supposed to occasion the disease. This cannot be the case, for it occurs very frequently when the ground is covered with snow. We are satisfied, although we may not succeed in satisfying the reader, that no one cause alone can produce the disease: there must be a diminution of vital energy, and this diminution may result, first, from poor diet. Dr. Graff tells us that the general appearance of these infected districts is somewhat peculiar. The quality of the soil is, in general, of an inferior description. The growth of timber is not observed to be so luxuriant as in situations otherwise similar, but is scrubby, and stunted in its perfect development, in many instances similating what in the west is denominated '*barrens.*'" We can easily conceive that these barrens do not furnish the proper amount of carbon (in the form of food) for the metamorphosis of the tissues; and if we take into consideration that the animal receives, during the day, while in search of this food, a large supply of oxygen, and at the same time the waste of the body is increased by the extra labor required to select sufficient nutriment, — it being scanty in such situations, — then it follows that this disproportion between the quantity of carbon in the food, and that of oxygen absorbed by the skin and lungs, must induce a diseased or abnormal condition. The animal is sometimes fat, at others lean. Some of the cows attacked with this disease were fat, and in apparent health, and nothing peculiar was observed until immediately preceding the outbreak of the fatal symptoms. The presence of fat is generally proof positive of an abnormal state; and in such cases the liver is often diseased; the blood then becomes loaded with fat and oil, and is finally deposited in the cellular tissues. The reader will now understand how an animal accumulates fat, notwithstanding it be furnished with insufficient diet. All that we wish to contend for is, that in such cases vital resistance is compromised. We have observed that, in the situation alluded to, vegetation was stunted, &c., and knowing that vegetables are composed of nearly the same materials which constitute animal organization, — the carbon or fat of the former being deposited in the seeds and fruits, and that of the latter in the cellular structure, — then we can arrive at but one conclusion, viz., that any location unfavorable to vegetation is likewise ill adapted to preserve the integrity of animal life.

In connection with this, it must be remembered that during the night the soil emits excrementitious vapors, which are taken into the animal system by the process of respiration. In the act of rumination, vapor is also enclosed in the globules of saliva, and thus reach the stomach. Many plants which during the day may be eaten with impunity by cattle, actually become poisonous during the night! This, we are aware, will meet with some opposition; to meet which we quote from Liebig: —

"How powerful, indeed, must the resistance appear which the vital force supplies to leaves charged with oil of turpentine or tannic acid, when we consider the affinity of oxygen for these compounds!

"This intensity of action, or of resistance, the plant obtains by means of the sun's light; the effect of which in chemical actions may be, and is, compared to that of a very high temperature, (moderate red heat.)

"During the night, an opposite process goes on in the plant; we see then that the constituents of the leaves and green parts combine with the oxygen of the air — a property which in daylight they did not possess.

"From these facts we can draw no other conclusion but this: that the intensity of the vital force diminishes with the abstraction of light; that, with the approach of night, a state of equilibrium is established; and that, in complete darkness, all those constituents of plants which, during the day, possessed the power of separating oxygen from chemical combinations, and of resisting its action, lose their power completely.

"A precisely similar phenomenon is observed in animals.

"The living animal body exhibits its peculiar manifestations of vitality only at certain temperatures. When exposed to a certain degree of cold, these vital phenomena entirely cease.

"The abstraction of heat must, therefore, be viewed as quite equivalent to a diminution of the vital energy; the resistance opposed by the vital force to external causes of disturbance must diminish, in certain temperatures, in the same ratio in which the tendency of the elements of the body to combine with the oxygen of the air increases."

Secondly. In the situations alluded to, we generally find poisonous and noxious plants, with an abundance of decayed vegetable matter. An English writer has said, "The farmers of England might advantageously employ a million at least of additional laborers in clearing their wide domains of noxious plants,* which would amply repay them in the superior quality of their produce. They would then feel the truth of that axiom in philosophy, "that he who can contrive to make two blades of grass, or wholesome grain, grow where one poisonous plant grew before, is a greater benefactor to the human race than all the conquerors or heroes who have ever lived." The noxious plants found in such abundance in the Western States are among the principal causes, either directly or indirectly, of the great mortality among men, horses, cattle, and sheep. The hay would be just as destructive as when in its green state, were it not that, in the process of drying, the volatile and poisonous properties of the buttercup, dandelion, poppy, and hundreds of similar destructive plants found in the hay, evaporate. It is evident that if animals have partaken of such plants, although death in all cases do not immediately follow, there must be a deficiency of vital resistance. or loss of equilibrium, and the animal is in a negative state. It is consequently obvious that when in such a state it is more liable to receive impressions from external agents — in short, is more subject to disease, and this disease may assume a definite form, regulated by location.

Thirdly A loss of vital resistance may result from drinking impure water. (See *Watering*, p. 15.) Dr. Graff tells us that "another peculiar appearance, which serves to distinguish these infected spots, is the breaking forth of numerous feeble springs, called oozes, furnishing but a trifling supply

* The American farmers are just beginning to wake up on this subject, and before long we hope to see our pasture lands free from all poisonous plants. Dr. Whitlaw says, "A friend of mine had two fields cleared of buttercups, dandelion, ox-eye, daisy, sorrel, hawk-weed, thistles, mullein, and a variety of other poisonous or noxious plants: they were dried, burnt, and their ashes strewed over the fields. He had them sown as usual, and found that the crops of hay and pasturage were more than double what they had been before. I was furnished with butter for two successive summers during the months of July and August of 1827. The butter kept for thirty days, and proved, at the end of that time, better than that fresh churned and brought to the Brighton or Margate markets. It would bear salting at that season of the year."

of water." Such water is generally considered unwholesome, and will, of course, deprive the system of its vital resistance, if partaken of.

Fourthly. A loss of vital resistance may result from exposure; for it is well known that cattle which have been regularly housed every night have escaped the attacks of this malady, and that when suffered to remain at large, they were frequently seized with it.

Lastly. The indirect causes of milk fever exist in any thing that can for a time prevent the free and full play of any part of the animal functions. The direct causes of death are chemical action, resulting from decomposition, which overcomes the vital principle.

Professor Liebig tells us, that "chemical action is opposed by the vital principle. The results produced depend upon the strength of their respective actions; either an equilibrium of both powers is attained, or the acting body yields to the superior force. If chemical action obtains the ascendency, it acts as a poison."

Remarks. — Let us suppose that one, or a combination of the preceding causes, has operated so as to produce an abnormal state in the system of a cow. She is then suffered to remain in the unhealthy district during the night: while there, exposed to the emanations from the soil, she requires the whole force of her vital energies to ward off chemical decompositions, and prevent encroachment on the various functions. A contest commences between the vital force and chemical action, and, after a hard conflict in their incessant endeavors to overcome each other, the chemical agency obtains the ascendency, and disease of a putrid type (milk fever) is the result. The disease may not immediately be recognized, for the process of decomposition may be insidious; yet the milk and flesh of such an animal may communicate the disease to man and other animals. It is well known that almost any part of animal bodies in a state of putrefaction, such as milk, cheese, muscle, pus, &c., communicate their own state of decomposition to other bodies. Many eminent medical men have lost their lives while dissecting, simply by putrefactive matter coming in contact with a slight wound or puncture. Dr. Graff made numerous experiments on dogs with the flesh, &c., of animals having died of milk sickness. He says, "My trials with the poisoned flesh were, for the most part, made on dogs, which I confined; and I often watched the effect of the poison when administered at regular intervals. In the space of forty-eight hours from the commencement of the administration of either the butter, cheese, or flesh, I have observed unequivocal appearances of their peculiar action, while the appetite remains unimpaired until the expiration of the fourth or fifth day." From the foregoing remarks, the reader will agree with us, that the disease is of a putrid type, and has a definite character. What is the reason of this definite character? All diseases are under the control of the immutable laws of nature. They preserve their identity in the same manner that races of men preserve theirs. Milk sickness of the malignant type luxuriates in the locations referred to, for the same reasons that yellow fever is peculiar to warm climates, and consumption to cold ones; and that different localities have distinct diseases; for example, ship fever, jail fever, &c.

Before disease can attack, and develop itself in the bodies of men or animals, the existing equilibrium of the vital powers must be disturbed; and the most common causes of this disturbance we have already alluded to. In reference to the milk, butter, cheese, &c., of infected animals, and their adaptation to develop disease in man, and in other locations than those referred to, we observe, that when a quantity, however small, of contagious matter is introduced into the stomach, if its antiseptic properties are the least deranged, the original disease (milk sickness) is produced, just as a small quantity of yeast will ferment a whole loaf. The transformation takes place through the medium of the blood, and produces a body identical with, or similar to, the exciting or contagious matter. The quantity of the latter must constantly augment; for the state of change or decomposition which affects one particle of the blood is imparted to others. The time necessary to accomplish it, however, depends on the amount of vital resistance, and of course varies in different animals. In process of time, the whole body becomes affected, and in like manner it is communicated to other individuals; and this may take place by simply respiring the carbonic acid gas, or morbific materials from the lungs, of diseased animals in the infected districts.

We are told that the latent condition of the disease may be discovered by subjecting the suspected animal to a violent degree of exercise. This is a precaution practised by butchers before slaughtering animals in any wise suspected of the poisonous contamination; * for according to the intensity of the existing cause, or its dominion over the vital power, it will be seized with tremors, spasms, convulsions, or even death. The reader is, probably, aware that an excess of mo-

* Unfortunately, they do not all practise it. Dr. Graff says, "There is a murderous practice now carried on in certain districts, in which the inhabitants will not themselves consume the butter and cheese manufactured; but, with little solicitude for the lives or health of others, they send it, in large quantities, to be sold in the cities of the west, particularly Louisville, Kentucky, and St. Louis, Missouri. Of the truth of this I am well apprised by actual observation; and I am as certain that it has often caused death in those cities, when the medical attendants viewed it as some anomalous form of disease, not suspecting the means by which poison had been conveyed among them. Physicians of the latter city, having been questioned particularly on this subject, have mentioned to me a singular and often fatal disease, which appeared in certain families, the cases occurring simultaneously, and all traces of it disappearing suddenly, and which I cannot doubt were the result of poisoned butter or cheese. This recklessness of human life it should be our endeavor to prevent; and the heartless wretches who practise it should be brought to suffer a punishment commensurate with the enormity of their crime. From the wide extent of the country in which it is carried on, we readily perceive the difficulties to be encountered in the effort to put a stop to the practice. This being the case, our next proper aim should be to investigate the nature of the cause, and establish a more proper plan of treatment, by which it may be robbed of its terrors, and the present large proportionate mortality diminished."

tion will sometimes cause instant death; for both men and animals, supposed to be in excellent health, are known to die suddenly from excessive labor. In some cases of excess of muscular exertion, the active force in living parts may be entirely destroyed in producing these violent mechanical results: hence we have a loss of equilibrium between voluntary and involuntary motion, and there is not sufficient vitality left to carry on the latter. Professor Liebig says, "A stag may be hunted to death. The condition of metamorphosis into which it has been brought by an enormous consumption both of force and of oxygen continues when all phenomena of motion have ceased, and the flesh becomes uneatable." A perfect equilibrium, therefore, between the consumption of vital force for the supply of waste, protecting the system from encroachments, and for mechanical effects, must exist; the animal is then in health: the contrary is obvious.

Treatment. — The greatest care must be taken to secure the patient good nutritious food, pure air, and water. The food should consist of a mixture of two or more of the following articles, which must be cooked: linseed, parsnips, shorts, carrots, meal, apples, barley, oats, turnips, slippery elm, oil cake, &c. We again remind the reader that no single or compound medicine can be procured that will be suitable for every stage of the disease; it must be treated according to its indications. Yet the following compound, aided by warmth, moisture, and friction, externally, will be found better than any medicine yet known. It consists of

Powdered charcoal, ...	8 ounces.
" sulphur, ...	2 ounces.
Fine salt, ...	3 ounces.
Oatmeal, ...	2 pounds.
Mandrake, (*podophyllum peltatum*,) . .	1 ounce.

After the ingredients are well mixed, divide the mass into fourteen parts, and give one night and morning.

Special Treatment with reference to the Symptoms. — Suppose the animal to be "off her feed," and the bowels are constipated; then give an aperient composed of

Extract of butternut, . . .	2 drachms.
Powdered capsicum, . . .	one third of a tea-spoonful.
Thoroughwort tea, . . .	2 quarts.

To be given at a dose, taking care to pour it down the throat in a gradual manner; for, if poured down too quick, it will fall into the paunch. If the rectum is suspected to be loaded with excrement, make use of the common soap-suds injection.

If the animal appears to walk about without any apparent object in view, there is reason to suppose that the brain is congested. This may be verified if the *sclerotica* (white of the eye) is of a deep red color. The following will be indicated: —

Mandrake, (*podophyllum peltatum*,)	1 table-spoonful.
Sulphur, ...	1 tea-spoonful.
Cream of tartar, ...	1 tea-spoonful.
Hot water, ...	2 quarts.

To be given at a dose. At the same time apply cold water to the head, and rub the spine and legs (below the knees) with the following counter-irritant: —

Powdered bloodroot or cayenne, . .	1 ounce.
" black pepper, ...	half an ounce.
Boiling vinegar, ...	1 quart.

Rub the mixture in while hot, with a piece of flannel.

If a trembling of the muscular system is observed, then give

Powdered ginger, ...	of each half a tea-spoonful.
" cinnamon, ...	
" golden seal, ...	

To be given at a dose, in half a gallon of catnip tea. Aid

the vital powers in producing a crisis by the warmth and moisture, as directed in the treatment of colds, &c.

It is necessary to keep the rectum empty by means of injections, forms of which will be found in this work.

The remedies we here recommend can be safely and successfully used by those unskilled in medicine; and, when aided by proper attention to the diet, ventilation, and comfort of the patient, we do not hesitate to say (provided, however, they are resorted to in the early stages) they will cure forty-nine cases out of fifty without the advice of a physician.

BONE DISORDER IN COWS.

WE have frequently seen accounts, in various papers, of "bone disorder in milch cows." The bony structure of animals is composed of vital solids studded with crystallizations of saline carbonates and phosphates, and is liable to take on morbid action similar to other textures. Disease of the bones may originate constitutionally, or from derangement of the digestive organs. We have, for example, *mollities ossium*, (softening of the bones;) the disease, however, is very rare. It may be known by the substance of the bones being soft and yielding, liable to bend with small force.

We have also *fragilitas ossium*, (brittleness of bones.) This is characterized by the bony system being of a friable nature, and liable to be fractured by slight force. We have in our possession the fragments of the small pastern of a horse, the bone having been broken into seventeen pieces, by a slight concussion, without any apparent injury to the skin and cellular substance; not the slightest external injury could be perceived.

There are several other diseases of the bones, which, we presume, our readers are acquainted with; such as *exostosis*, *caries*, &c., neither of which apply to the malady under consideration. We merely mention these for the purpose of showing that the bones are not exempt from disease, any more than other structures; yet it does not always follow that a lack of the phosphate of lime in cow's milk is a sure sign of diseased bones.

Reader, we do not like the term "*bone disorder:*" it does not throw the least light on the nature of the malady; it savors too much of "*horn ail,*" "*tail ail*" — terms which only apply to symptoms. We are told also that, in this disease, "*the bones threaten to cave in — have wasted away.*" If they do threaten to cave in, the best way we know of to give them an outward direction is, to promote the healthy secretions and excretions by a well-regulated diet, and to stimulate the digestive organs to healthy action. If the bones "have wasted away," we should like to have a few of them in our collection of morbid anatomy. That the bones should waste away, and be capable of assuming their original shape simply by feeding bone meal, is something never dreamt of in our philosophy.* Besides, if the cows get well, (we are told they do,) then we must infer that the bones possess the properties of sudden expansion and contraction, similar to those of the muscles. It may be well for us to observe, that not only the bones, but all parts of animal organization, expand and contract in an imperceptible manner. Thus, up to the period of puberty, all parts expand: old age comes on, and with it a gradual wasting and collapse. This is a natural result — one of the uncompromising laws of nature, over which human agency (bone meal included) has not the least control. If the bones are diseased, it results either from impaired digestion or a disproportion between the carbon of the food and the oxygen respired; hence the "bone disorder," not being persistent, is only a result — a symptom; and as such we view it. As far as we have been able to ascertain the nature of the malady, as manifested by the symptoms, (*caving in*, *wasting*, *absence of phosphate of lime in the milk*, &c.,) we give it as our opinion, — and we think our medical brethren will agree with us, (although we do not often agree,) — that "bone disorder" is a symptom of a disease very prostrating in its character, originating in the digestive organs; hence not confined to the bones, but affecting all parts of the animal more or less. And the only true plan of treatment consists in restoring healthy action to the whole

* Whenever there is a deficiency of carbon, bone meal may assist to support combustion in the lungs, and by that means restore healthy action of the different functions, provided, however, the digestive organs, aided by the vital power, can overcome the chemical action by which the atoms of bone meal are held together.

animal system. The ways and means of accomplishing this object are various. If it is clearly ascertained that the animal system is deficient in phosphate of lime, we see no good reason why bone meal should not be included among our remedial agents; yet, as corn meal and linseed contain a large amount of phosphate, we should prefer them to bone dust, although we do not seriously object to its use.

The value of food or remedial agents consists in their adaptation to assimilation; in other words, an absence of chemical properties. These may be very complex; yet, if they are only held together by a weak chemical action, they readily yield to the vital principle, and are transformed. Atoms of bones are held together by a strong chemical affinity; and the vital principle, in order to convert bone dust into component parts of the organism, must employ more force to transform them than it would require for the same purpose when corn meal or linseed were used, their chemical affinity being weaker than that of bones.

In the treatment of any disease, we always endeavor to ascertain its causes, and, if possible, remove them; and whatever may be indicated we endeavor to supply to the system. Thus, if phosphates were indicated, we should use them. In cases of general debility, however, we should prefer linseed or corn meal, aided by stimulants, to bone dust. Why not use the bone dust for manure? The animal would then have the benefit of it in its fodder.

In reference to a deficiency of phosphate of lime in the milk, we would observe, that it may result either from impaired digestion, (in such cases, a large amount of that article may be expelled from the system in the form of excrements,) or the food may lack it. We then have a sick plant, for we believe that the phosphate of lime is as necessary for the growth of the plant as it seems to be for animal development. If the plant lacks this important constituent, then its vitality, as a whole, will be impaired. This is all we desire to contend for in the animal, viz., that the disease s general, and cannot be considered or treated as a local affection.

It has been observed that successive cultivation exhausts the soil, and deprives it of the constituents necessary for vegetable development. If so, it follows that there will be a deficiency of silecia, carbonate of lime, — in short, a loss of carbon, hydrogen, nitrogen, and oxygen, not of phosphate of lime alone.

The fields might be made to produce the requisite amount of nutriment by replacing every year, in the form of animal excrement, straw, wood-ashes, and charcoal, as much as we remove from them in the form of produce. An increase of crop can only be obtained when we add more to the soil than we take away from it.

"In Flanders, the yearly loss of the necessary matters in the soil is completely restored by covering the fields with ashes of wood or bones, which may, or may not, have been lixiviated. The great importance of manuring with ashes has been long recognized by agriculturists as the result of experience. So great a value, indeed, is attached to this material in the vicinity of Marburg, and in the Wetterau, — two well-known agricultural districts, — that it is transported, as a manure, from the distance of eighteen or twenty-four miles. Its use will be at once perceived, when it is considered that the ashes, after being washed with water, contain silicate of potass exactly in the same proportion as in the straw, and that their only other constituents are salts of phosphoric acid."

It is well known that phosphate of lime, potass, silecia, carbonate of lime, magnesia, and soda are discharged in the excrement and urine of the cow; and this happens when they are not adapted to assimilation as well as when present in excess. If it is clearly proved that the bones of a cow are weak, then we should be inclined to prescribe phosphates; if they are brittle, we should prescribe gelatinous preparations; but not in the form of bone dust: we should use linseed, which is known to be rich in phosphates. At the same time, the general health must be improved.

It is well known that some cows cannot be fattened, although they have an abundance of the best kind of fodder In such cases, we find the digestive organs deranged, which disturbs the equilibrium of the whole animal economy. The food may then be said to be a direct cause of disease.

The effects of insufficient food are well known; debility includes them all. If there is not sufficient carbon in the food, the animal is deprived of the power of reproducing itself, and the cure consists in supplying the deficiency. At the same time, every condition of nutrition should be considered; and if the function of digestion is impaired, we must look to those of absorption, circulation, and secretion also, for they will be more or less involved. If the appetite is impaired, accompanied by a loss of cud, it shows that the stomach is overloaded, or that its function is suspended: stimulants and tonics are then indicated. A voracious appetite indicates the presence of morbid accumulations in the stomach and bowels, and they should be cleansed by aperients; after which, a change of diet will generally effect a cure. When gas accumulates in the intestines, we have evidence of a loss of vital power in the digestive organs; fermentation takes place before the food can be digested.

The cure consists in restoring the lost function. Diarrhœa is generally caused by exposure, (taking cold,) or by eating poisons and irritating substances; the cure may be accomplished by removing the cold, and cleansing the system of the irritants. Costiveness often arises from the absorption of the fluids from the solids in their slow progress through the intestines; exercise will then be indicated. An occasional injection, however, may be given, if necessary. General debility, we have said, may arise from insufficient food; to which we may add the popular practice of milking the cow while pregnant, much of which milk is yielded at the hazard of her own health and that of her fœtus. Whatever is taken away from the cow in the form of milk ought to be replaced by the food. Proper attention, however, must be paid to the state of the digestive organs: they must not be overtaxed with indigestible substances. With this object in view, we recommend a mixed diet; for no animal can subsist on a single article of food. Dogs die, although fed on jelly; they cannot live upon white bread, sugar, or starch, if these are given as food, to the exclusion of all other substances. Neither can a horse or cow live on hay alone: they will, sooner or later, give evidences of disease. They require stimulants. Common salt is a good stimulant. This explains why salt hay should be occasionally fed to milch cows; it not only acts as a stimulant, but is also an antiseptic, preventing putrefaction, &c.

A knowledge of the constituents of milk may aid the farmer in selecting the substances proper for the nourishment of animals, and promotive of the lacteal secretion; for much of the food contains those materials united, though not always in the same form. "The constituents of milk are cheese, or caseine — a compound containing nitrogen in large proportion; butter, in which hydrogen abounds; and sugar of milk, a substance with a large quantity of hydrogen and oxygen in the same proportions as in water. It also contains, in solution, lactate of soda, phosphate of lime, (the latter in very small quantities,) and common salt; and a peculiar aromatic product exists in the butter, called butyric acid." — *Liebig.*

It is very difficult to explain the changes which the food undergoes in the animal laboratory, (the stomach,) because that organ is under the dominion of the vital force — an immaterial agency which the chemist cannot control. Yet we are justified in furnishing the animal with the elements of its own organization; for although they may not be deposited in the different structures in their original atoms, they may be changed into other compounds, somewhat similar. Liebig tells us that whether the elements of non-azotized food take an inmediate share in the act of transformation of tissues, or whether their share in that process be an indirect one, is a question probably capable of being resolved by careful and cautious experiment and observation. It is possible that these constituents of food, after undergoing some change, are carried from the intestinal canal directly to the liver, and that there they are converted into bile, where they meet with the products of the metamorphosed tissues, and subsequently complete their course through the circulation.

This opinion appears more probable, when we reflect that as yet no trace of starch or sugar has been detected in arterial blood, not even in animals that have been fed exclusively with these substances.

The following tables, from Liebig's Chemistry, will give the reader the difference between what is taken into the system and what passes out.

FOOD CONSUMED BY A COW IN TWENTY-FOUR HOURS.

Articles of food.	Weight in the fresh state.	Weight in the dry state.	Carbon.	Hydrogen.	Oxygen.	Nitrogen.	Salts and earthy matters.
Potatoes,	15000	4170	1839.0	241.9	1830.6	50.0	208.5
After grass,	7500	6315	2974.4	353.6	2204.0	151.5	631.5
Water,	60000	—	—	—	—	—	50.0
Total,	82500	10485	4813.4	595.5	4034.6	201.5	889.0

EXCRETIONS OF A COW IN TWENTY-FOUR HOURS.

Excretions.	Weight in the fresh state.	Weight in the dry state.	Carbon.	Hydrogen.	Oxygen.	Nitrogen.	Salts and earthy matters.
Excrements,	28413	4000.0	1712.0	208.0	1508.0	92.0	480.0
Urine,	8200	960.8	261.4	25.0	253.7	36.5	384.2
Milk,	8539	1150.6	628.2	99.0	321.0	46.0	56.4
Total,	45152	6111.4	2601.6	332.0	2082.7	174.5	920.6
Total of first part of this table,	82500	10485.0	4813.4	595.5	4034.6	201.5	889.0
Difference,	37348	4374.6	2211.8	263.5	1951.9	27.0	31.6

FOOD CONSUMED BY A HORSE IN TWENTY-FOUR HOURS.

Articles of food.	Weight in the fresh state.	Weight in the dry state.	Carbon.	Hydrogen.	Oxygen.	Nitrogen.	Salts and earthy matters.
Hay,	7500	6465	2961.0	323.2	2502.0	97.0	581.8
Oats,	2270	1927	977.0	123.3	707.2	42.4	77.1
Water,	16000	—	—	—	—	—	13.3
Total,	25770	8392	3938.0	446.5	3209.2	139.4	672.2

EXCRETIONS OF A HORSE IN TWENTY-FOUR HOURS.

Excretions.	Weight in the fresh state.	Weight in the dry state.	Carbon.	Hydrogen.	Oxygen.	Nitrogen.	Salts and earthy matters.
Urine,	1330	302	108.7	11.5	34.1	37.8	109.9
Excrements,	14250	3525	1364.4	179.8	1328.9	77.6	574.6
Total,	15580	3827	1472.9	191.3	1363.0	115.4	684.5
Total of first part of this table,	25770	8392	3938.0	446.5	3209.2	139.4	672.2
Difference,	10190	4565	2465.1	255.2	1846.2	24.0	12.3

The weights in these tables are given in grammes. 1 gramme is equal to 15.44 grains Troy, very nearly.

It will be seen from these tables that a large proportion of carbon, hydrogen, oxygen, nitrogen, and earthy matters are again returned to the soil. From this we infer that more of these matters being present in the food than were requisite for the purpose of assimilation, they were removed from the system in the form of excrement. Two suggestions here present themselves for the consideration of the farmer, viz., that the manure increases in value in proportion to the richness of food, and that more of the latter is often given to a cow than is necessary for the manufacture of healthy chyle.

In view, then, of preventing "bone disorder," which we have termed *indigestion*, we should endeavor to ascertain what articles are best for food, and learn, from the experience of others, what have been universally esteemed as such, and, by trying them on our own animals, prove whether we actually find them so. Scalded or boiled food is better adapted to the stomach of animals than food otherwise prepared, and is so much less injurious. The agents that act on the internal system are those which, in quantities sufficient for an ordinary meal, supply the animal system with stimulus and nutriment just enough for its wants, and contain nothing in their nature inimical to the vital operations. All such articles are properly termed food. (For treatment, see *Hide-bound*, p. 196.)